Neuroanatomy Made Easy and Understandable

Third Edition

by

Michael Liebman, Ph.D.
The Hebrew University-Hadassah Medical School
Jerusalem

and

former Professorial Lecturer in Anatomy
Department of Anatomy
The George Washington University Medical School
Washington, D.C.

with a contribution by

Rina Tadmor, M.D.
Head of the Neuroradiology Section
Sheba Medical Center-Tel Hashomer
Tel-Aviv University Medical School

AN ASPEN PUBLICATION®
Aspen Publishers, Inc.   1986   Rockville, Maryland
Royal Tunbridge Wells

Aspen Publishers, Inc.
1600 Research Boulevard
Rockville, Maryland 20850

Manufactured in the United States of America

Library of Congress Cataloging in Publication Data

Liebman, Michael

Neuroanatomy made easy and understandable.

Includes index.
1. Neuroanatomy. I. Tadmor, Rina, II. Title.
[DNLM: 1. Nervous system–Anatomy and histology. WL 101 L716n]
QM451.L53   1986   611'.8   86-17332
ISBN 0-87189-396-7

This book is dedicated to my parents and teachers

Table of Contents

Don't Skip This Introduction

Today you are faced with the problem of having to know more and more material in a shorter and shorter period of time. With neuroanatomy this problem is compounded because it is one of the most difficult subjects to grasp. Most "neuro" texts are very broad in scope and crammed with seemingly endless details, the latest theories, and so on. At this stage, however, you're unable to separate the wheat from the chaff; that is, to distinguish what is important for you from what is not. Consequently, you usually try to learn it all because you are afraid something will appear on the exam that you didn't read up on. Under conditions of high pressure and little time, this usually results in a monumental effort of memory, accompanied by little understanding and retention.

In this book I have cut out the fat of extraneous details, theories, and the like, and left *the essentials that form the basis of neuroanatomy, neurophysiology, neuropharmacology, physical diagnosis, and neurology, and for passing exams.* Although the subject is presented in a deceptively simple, breezy, and personal style, you must not assume that this was done by sacrificing material. The main reason for this approach was to make the subject easier to read, understand, and retain. Therefore, once you know the material in this book, you will be able to read and quickly understand more detailed neuroanatomy texts and reference books, should the need arise.

The terminology can throw you for two reasons. First, it is often redundant. For example, a group of nerve fibers may be called a tract, fasciculus, column, lemniscus, funiculus, or bundle—all terms accepted and used by the medical and scientific community. Second, the terminology is full of weird-sounding names of Greek and Latin origins. As for the first, the author obviously cannot at his whim cut out recognized terms, but he can point out those that are synonymous. As for the second problem, I have prepared a special glossary that not only explains the meaning and origin of the names, but also lists a common everyday word derived from them. For example, *fornix* is a Latin word meaning an arch and is applied to a curved bundle of nerve fibers. The related everyday word is fornication, and the reason for this is that in ancient Rome the prostitutes used to hang around the arches of the aqueducts!

I strongly recommend that you read each chapter before going to each lecture; then, instead of furiously trying to write down every word, you'll be able to sit back, absorb, and understand the material and leisurely jot down additional notes and drawings.

This third edition contains a new appendix of normal and pathologic magnetic resonance imaging (MRI) scans and a new relaxing "Did You Know" section. More pathologic CT scans have been added, and most chapters have been expanded by the addition of clinical facts that show the importance of the basic material presented here.

Finally, I would welcome and appreciate suggestions and criticisms.
Good luck!

Chapter 1

The Microscopic Basis of Neuroanatomy

The basic unit of the nervous system, as in all other systems of the body, is the cell, which here is called the *neuron*. The main properties that distinguish neurons from other types of cells are their specialization for conduction of impulses, their great sensitivity to oxygen deprivation, their importance for many vital functions, and the fact that they don't multiply. (It is this last fact that is responsible for so many of the incurable conditions that you will see—paralysis, chronic vegetative states, palsy, blindness, etc.) This text discusses many types of neurons, and they all have the above-mentioned characteristics.

A typical neuron (Figure 1) consists of a cell body with a large *nucleus* that has a dark central *nucleolus*. Fine particles, known as *Nissl granules*, are scattered throughout most of the cytoplasm. Projecting from the cell body are many short processes—the *dendrites*—which receive impulses from other neurons and conduct them to the cell body. From the cell body a single long process—the *axon*—conducts the nerve impulse away and out to the dendrites of other neurons and to muscles and glands.

The site of contact between the axon of one neuron and the dendrites of another is the *synapse*, and the site of contact between an axon and a muscle fiber is the *motor end plate*. However, the impulse does not pass directly from neuron to neuron or neuron to muscle. Rather, it is transmitted by chemical mediators called *neurotransmitters*. The most widespread of these is *acetylcholine*; others include epinephrine, dopamine, and gamma-aminobutyric acid (GABA). The basic mechanism is as follows: the nervous impulse, which is measurable with fine instruments, travels down the axon until it reaches the synapse. Here it causes the release of neurotransmitter from the end of the axon, and this passes through the ultramicroscopic synaptic gap to the adjacent dendrites, where it triggers a new impulse that is then propagated in the second neuron (Figure 1). A single axon may synapse with the dendrites of several or even hundreds of neurons, and the dendrites of one nerve cell can receive impulses from the axons of many neurons. Finally, there can be a combination of these two situations (Figure 2).

The axons of nearly all neurons are covered with a fatty white substance called *myelin*; in order for most impulses to be propagated, myelin must be present. In infants, myelin has not yet been laid down completely, and the completion of this process is one of the factors in the development of walking. In certain diseases, such as multiple sclerosis, the myelin degenerates and the patient suffers from a loss of various sensations and/or a diminution of movements. The process of *myelinization* (laying down of myelin) is performed by special cells that form an outer enveloping layer around the axon. This layer is known as the *sheath of Schwann* (*neurolemma*). Myelin is not a continuous layer but has gaps—the *nodes of Ranvier*—and here the overlying sheath of Schwann dips down and comes in contact with the axon (Figure 1).

Functionally and structurally there are many kinds of neurons; several of the most common are shown in Figure 3. A *motor* or *efferent neuron* is one that transmits impulses to muscles and/or glands, whereas a *sensory* or *afferent neuron* propagates sensory impulses. The nervous tissue of the brain and spinal cord is divided into *gray matter*, which is composed mostly of nerve cell bodies, and *white matter*, which is made up of the white axon fibers. Furthermore, nervous tissue has special cells—the *glia*—which are divided into three types: first are the *microglia*, which act as scavengers (*phagocytes*); the second are the *oligodendroglia*. Because the axons within the spinal cord and brain do not have a sheath of Schwann, it is thought that the oligodendroglia in these areas lay down the myelin. The third type of glia cells are *astrocytes*, whose functions are to hold together the delicate neurons and to help create the blood-brain barrier.

It's known that most substances that leave the capillaries to enter the surrounding tissues are unable to penetrate the capillaries of the central nervous system (CNS). This unique "barrier" is known as the blood-brain barrier. Oxygen, carbon dioxide, amino acids, a few sugars, and many lipid soluble substances, such as general anesthetics, can pass the barrier, but most high-molecular weight substances, most sugars, and most protein-bound substances can't penetrate the CNS capillaries. It is generally accepted that this barrier is caused by

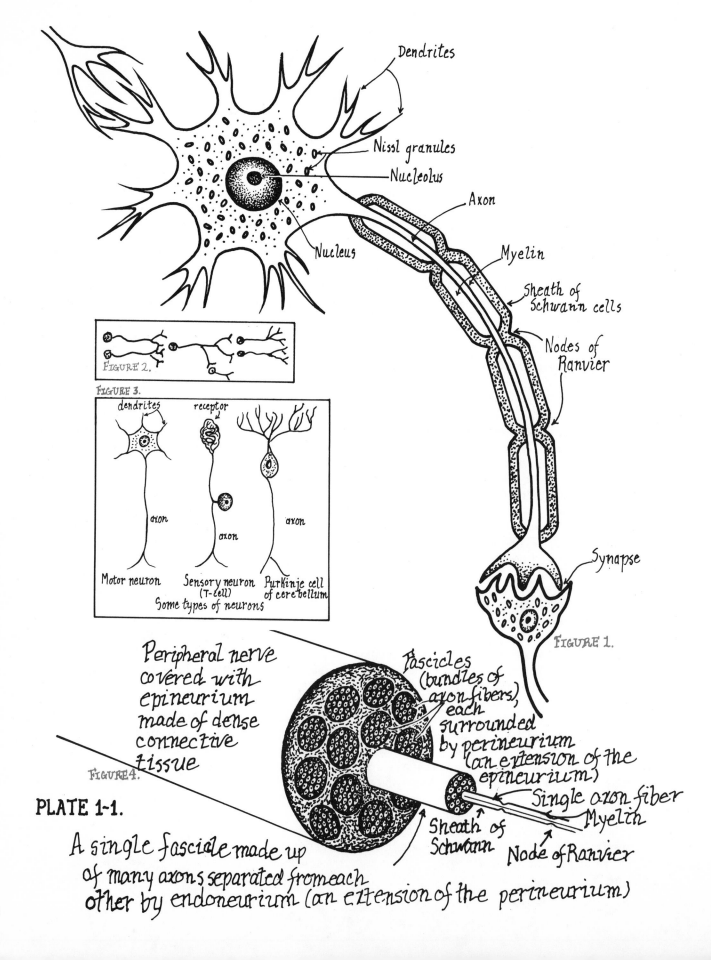

Dendrites

Nissl granules

Nucleolus

Axon

Myelin

Sheath of Schwann cells

Nodes of Ranvier

Nucleus

Synapse

FIGURE 2.

FIGURE 3.

dendrites

receptor

axon

axon

axon

Motor neuron

Sensory neuron (T-cell)

Purkinje cell of cerebellum

Some types of neurons

FIGURE 1.

Peripheral nerve covered with epineurium made of dense connective tissue

FIGURE 4.

Fascicles (bundles of axon fibers), each surrounded by perineurium (an extension of the epineurium)

Single axon fiber

Myelin

Node of Ranvier

Sheath of Schwann

PLATE 1-1.

A single fascicle made up of many axons separated from each other by endoneurium (an extension of the perineurium)

2

two factors. First, the astrocytes have pseudopodia-like extensions that surround and envelop the outer wall of the capillaries, thus effectively sealing them off. Second, the endothelial borders of the CNS capillaries—in contrast to all other capillaries in the body—form tight junctions with each other.

In addition to neurons and glia, there are the *ependymal cells* that line the central canal of the spinal cord as well as the *ventricles*, and which are the first cells to appear during the embryonic development of the nervous system.

Although the nerve pathways in the figures in other chapters are represented by a single axon, this is artistic license for the sake of clarity. In reality every nerve and pathway is made up of many bundles, called *fascicles*, which in turn are made up of hundreds and hundreds of axons (Figure 4).

CLINICAL ASPECTS

Because mature neurons do not multiply, they are unable to give rise to brain tumors. The great majority of *neoplasms* (tumors) of the nervous system arise from glial cells or from the proliferation of other tissue cells found in conjunction with the brain, such as connective tissue or the epithelial cells of the pituitary gland. Very rarely, neurons still in an immature state give rise to tumors known as *neuroblastomas*.

When a nerve is cut, a series of characteristic reactions takes place. That part of the axon distal to the injury quickly breaks down and dies in a process known as *Wallerian degeneration*. The section of axon still attached to the cell body initially undergoes some degeneration, but if the damage isn't too extensive, it will start growing. However, its growth is inhibited by the rapid proliferation of Schwann cells, which form a dense scar-like mass. In cases where the epineural layer of the severed ends of a peripheral nerve is sewn back together, growth will occur and there will be some renewal of normal function. The amount of renewal depends on such factors as the degree and location of injury, the quickness and skill of repair, the amount of glial cell proliferation at the repaired site, and the age of the patient. Unfortunately, axons within the brain and spinal cord cannot grow if they are severely damaged or cut.

Multiple sclerosis (MS) is a fairly common neurologic disease that attacks primarily young adults in the 20–40 age group but never children under 10 or adults over 60. The myelin in the CNS breaks down, producing a variety of symptoms, such as a reduction or loss of sensation, muscle weakness or fatigue, numbness or tingling in the extremities, vertigo, or diplopia (double vision). Indeed *the variety and mixture of symptoms is one of the most important clues in diagnosing the illness*. The cause of the disease is unknown, and at the present time there is no known cure or means of prevention. Strangely, the myelin often forms again, and the symptoms disappear until the myelin degenerates once again. A patient may have a few such episodes and then recover completely, or the attacks may progress and spread rapidly, ending in death. In many other individuals the attacks and remissions last for many years.

One of the most puzzling things about multiple sclerosis is that in tropical areas the incidence of the illness is 1 per 100,000, whereas in colder areas, such as Canada and Northern Europe, the incidence soars to 30–80 per 100,000. Epidemiologic studies in Israel, a subtropical country that has received waves of immigrants from around the world, have been revealing. Those individuals who came from cold countries and were past the age of puberty had the same incidence of MS as persons in their country of origin, whereas those from cold countries who came before puberty while their thymuses were still large and active had the low rate of incidence characteristic of inhabitants of warm climates. The explanation for this fact may hold the key to the cause and cure of the disease.

Until recently it was difficult to make a final diagnosis of MS because there were no laboratory examinations for it. But now using magnetic resonance imaging (MRI), the degenerating plaques of myelin are easily seen (Appendix IV, Figure 8), thus quickly confirming the tentative diagnosis.

Chapter 2

The Macroscopic Basis of Neuroanatomy

This chapter deals with the macroscopic, many-named areas of the brain—a topic that can be very boring. However, it is necessary because one can't proceed with the study of the nervous pathways without knowing where they start, through what structures they pass, and where they end.

The nervous system is divided arbitrarily into a central and a peripheral part. The *central nervous system* (CNS) consists of the *brain* and the *spinal cord*. The *peripheral nervous system* is made up of the 12 pairs of cranial nerves and all the remaining nerves of the body and their associated collections of cell bodies—the *ganglia*.

FIVE PARTS OF THE BRAIN

The brain is divided on an embryologic basis into five parts: *telencephalon, diencephalon, mesencephalon, pons* and *cerebellum*, and the *medulla oblongata*. In this chapter we consider these five parts one by one.

Telencephalon

The telencephalon is the center for the highest functions and is therefore the most developed in humans. It is composed of two major structures: the *cerebral hemispheres* and the *basal ganglia*. The latter, which are the areas for crude motor activity, are buried deep in the cerebral hemispheres and can only be seen when the brain is cut. The cerebral hemispheres, on the other hand, are two very large structures divided from each other by the *median longitudinal fissure* and comprise most of the brain matter that is seen (Figure 1).* Their convex surface is made up of convolutions called *gyri*, which are separated from each other by shallow grooves—the *sulci* (a deep sulcus is called a fissure). Although certain gyri and sulci are present in almost every human brain, no two brains or even hemispheres of the same brain have exactly the same pattern of gyri and sulci. Two grooves, the lateral *fissure* and the *central sulcus*, help divide each hemisphere into four main areas, or *lobes* (Figure 2). The *frontal lobe*

is anterior to the central sulcus, and the *parietal lobe* is posterior to it (Figure 2). Lying below the *lateral fissure* is the *temporal lobe*, and an imaginary line drawn down from the *parieto-occipital fissure* separates the parietal lobe from the *occipital lobe* (Figure 2). As if there weren't enough divisions already, each lobe has its specific areas and gyri. For example, in the frontal lobe the *precentral gyrus*, lying just anterior to the central sulcus, is the motor center that initiates impulses to the voluntary muscles. The most anterior area, the *frontal pole*, is the seat of personality (Figure 3). Injuries here often result in alterations of personality. These and other areas are discussed later in great detail.

The telencephalon also occupies much of the base of the brain. Here are situated the *orbital gyri*, and resting on them are found the *olfactory nerves*, which are the nerves of smell, and the *optic nerves*, which transmit visual impulses from the eye to the brain (Figure 4). The optic nerves converge on each other, cross at the *chiasma*, and then proceed posteriorly as the *optic tracts* (Figure 4). This view of the telencephalon also reveals the *parahippocampal gyrus* of the temporal pole with its characteristic bulge, the *uncus*.

When the brain is cut in a horizontal plane, one sees that the cerebral hemispheres have an outer gray layer, the *cortex*, which is composed primarily of cell bodies, and an inner white mass made up of myelinated axons (Figure 5). Axons that pass from one hemisphere to the other are called *commissural fibers*; the best example is the large *corpus callosum* (Figures 5 and 6). Long and short *associative fibers* are those that pass from lobe to lobe or from gyrus to gyrus in the same hemisphere. Finally, those axons that ascend to or descend from the cerebral hemisphere to other areas of the CNS are called *projection fibers*, and most are situated in the *internal capsule*. This structure has an *anterior limb*, a *posterior limb*, and a section between the two called the *genu* (Figure 5). Just lateral to the genu are located some of the *basal ganglia*; for example, the globus pallidus and the putamen (Figure 5).

Some neuroanatomy texts maintain that there are five lobes of the brain, whereas others claim there are six. If the lateral fissure is spread apart, one sees the *insula*, which is an unfolding of the

---

*In addition to the drawings in this chapter and in Appendix II, the reader should refer to the CT scans in Figures 1–5 in Appendix III and to the MRI scans in Appendix IV.

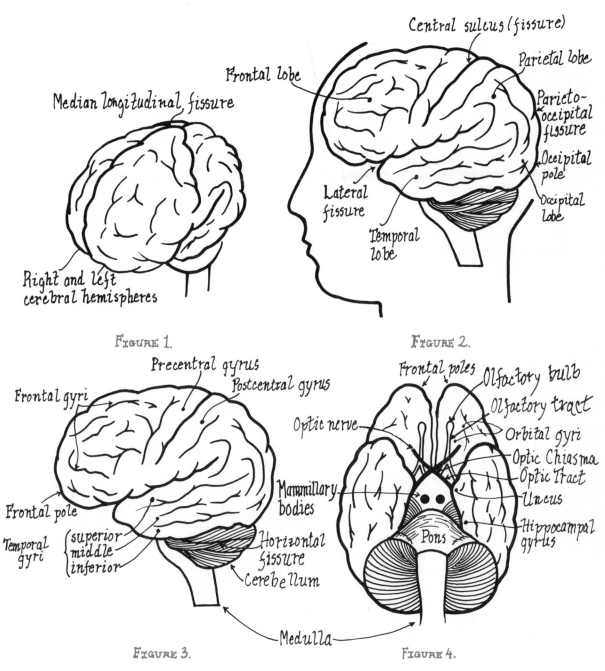

Median longitudinal fissure

Right and left cerebral hemispheres

FIGURE 1.

Central sulcus (fissure)

Frontal lobe

Parietal lobe

Parieto-occipital fissure

Occipital pole

Occipital lobe

Lateral fissure

Temporal lobe

FIGURE 2.

Frontal gyri

Precentral gyrus

Postcentral gyrus

Frontal pole

Temporal gyri

superior
middle
inferior

Horizontal fissure

Cerebellum

FIGURE 3.

Frontal poles

Optic nerve

Mammillary bodies

Olfactory bulb

Olfactory tract

Orbital gyri

Optic Chiasma

Optic Tract

Uncus

Hippocampal gyrus

Pons

FIGURE 4.

Medulla

PLATE 2~1.

5

cerebral hemisphere. The insula has no known function in humans and is considered a fifth lobe. The cerebral cortex of the frontal, parietal, and temporal lobes surrounding the lateral fissure is known as the *operculum*. The limbic, or sixth lobe, is made up of the *cingulate, parahippocampal,* and *dentate gyri*. (The author is waiting for the discovery of a seventh and maybe even an eighth lobe.)

Diencephalon

The diencephalon is the second division of the brain. It is a small area situated between the cerebral hemispheres and is seen best on a midsagittal view (Figure 6). The diencephalon is divided into the *thalamus*, which is the main relay center for the nervous system, and, below it, the *hypothalamus* (Figure 6). The hypothalamus is a vital area concerned with temperature control, emotional states, and control over the autonomic nervous system. In addition, the diencephalon is made up of the *medial* and *lateral geniculate bodies*, the *subthalamic nucleus*, and the *pineal body*. (Plates IV and IX in Appendix II, "Atlas of the Brain").

Mesencephalon

The mesencephalon, the pons, and the medulla oblongata together form a wedge-shaped structure, the *brainstem*, which extends down from the base of the brain to the *foramen magnum* of the skull (Figure 6). The mesencephalon, or *midbrain*, is the smallest of the five divisions of the brain and is located between the diencephalon and the pons (Figure 6). The area above the *aqueduct of Sylvius* (cerebral aqueduct) is the *tectum*, which is made up of four rounded projections—the *corpora quadrigemina*. The upper two projections form the *superior colliculi*, and the lower two the *inferior colliculi*. In the body or *tegmentum* of the midbrain pass various fiber tracts. Also situated there are the *red nucleus*, the *oculomotor nerve* and its nucleus, and the *trochlear nerve* and its nucleus. At the base of the midbrain there is a pair of huge fiber bundles, the *crus cerebri* (or *basis pedunculi*), which is a continuation of the descending projection fibers of the internal capsule (Figure 6a). Finally, situated between the tegmentum and the crus cerebri is the *substantia nigra*. The latter plus the crus and tegmentum make up the *cerebral peduncle*.

Pons and Cerebellum

The pons and cerebellum together make up the fourth division of the brain (Figures 6 and 7). The cerebellum is a many-folded structure located under the occipital lobe and is concerned with equilibrium, muscle tone, and the coordination of muscle activity.

The names of the subdivisions and fissures of the cerebellum are very numerous, but only the important ones are mentioned here and in the figures. The *archicerebellum* is the oldest part of the cerebellum and is made up of the central nodulus and the paired flocculus. Together they form the *flocculonodular* lobe (Figure 7), which is concerned with equilibrium. The *paleocerebellum* is an old part of the cerebellum composed of the anterior lobe and part of the vermis and is primarily concerned with muscle tone (Figure 7). The newest and largest part of the cerebellum is the *neocerebellum*, which is made up of the posterior lobe and most of the vermis (Figure 7) and which deals with the coordination (synergy) of voluntary muscle activity. Four important nuclei, the *Dentate, Emboliborm, Fastigial,* and *Globus* (DEFG) are also situated within the cerebellum.

Passing between the cerebellum and the underlying brainstem are three pairs of fiber bundles: the

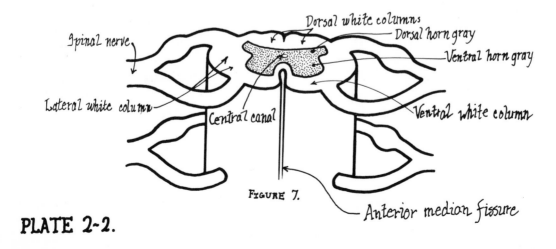

PLATE 2-2.

FIGURE 7.

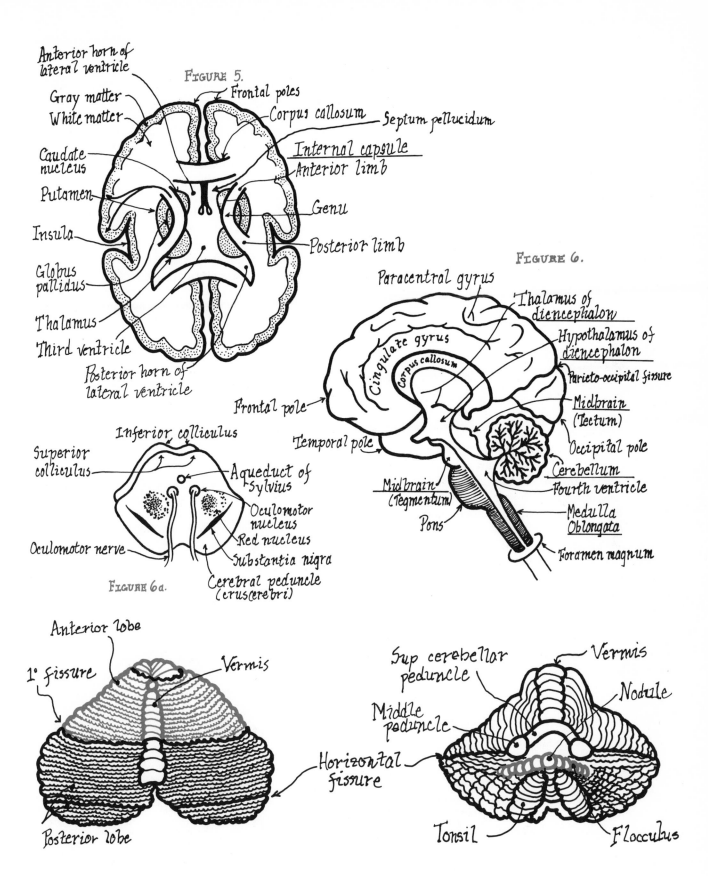

FIGURE 5.

Anterior horn of lateral ventricle
Gray matter
White matter
Caudate nucleus
Putamen
Insula
Globus pallidus
Thalamus
Third ventricle
Posterior horn of lateral ventricle

Frontal poles
Corpus callosum
Septum pellucidum
Internal capsule
Anterior limb
Genu
Posterior limb

FIGURE 6.

Paracentral gyrus
Cingulate gyrus
Corpus callosum
Thalamus of diencephalon
Hypothalamus of diencephalon
Parieto-occipital fissure
Midbrain (Tectum)
Occipital pole
Cerebellum
Fourth ventricle
Frontal pole
Temporal pole
Midbrain (Tegmentum)
Pons
Medulla Oblongata
Foramen magnum

Superior colliculus
Inferior colliculus
Aqueduct of Sylvius
Oculomotor nucleus
Red nucleus
Substantia nigra
Cerebral peduncle (crus cerebri)
Oculomotor nerve

FIGURE 6a.

Anterior lobe
1° fissure
Vermis
Horizontal fissure
Posterior lobe

Sup cerebellar peduncle
Middle peduncle
Horizontal fissure
Vermis
Nodule
Tonsil
Flocculus

FIGURE 7a. Superior surface of cerebellum

FIGURE 7b. Inferior surface of cerebellum

PLATE 2~3

7

superior, middle, and *inferior cerebellar peduncles* (see Chapter 11). They are also known as the *brachium conjunctivum,* the *brachium pontis,* and the *restiform body,* respectively. The pons is located between the midbrain and the medulla and is separated from the overlying cerebellum by a cavity—the *fourth ventricle* (Figure 6). Through the pons pass various ascending and descending fiber tracts. Also in the pons are the nuclei of the fifth cranial nerve (*trigeminal nerve*), the sixth cranial nerve (*abducens nerve*), and the seventh cranial nerve (*facial nerve*).

Medulla Oblongata

The medulla oblongata is the last division of the brain. It becomes continuous with the spinal cord at the foramen magnum (Figure 6). Like the pons and midbrain, it contains ascending and descending fiber tracts, as well as the nuclei of cranial nerves VIII through XII. The respiratory and cardiac centers are also situated in the medulla.

SPINAL CORD

The spinal cord is a long cylindrical structure beginning at the foramen magnum and descending in the vertebral canal to about the level of the second lumbar vertebra (L_2). The cord serves as the main pathway (highway) for the ascending and descending fibers tracts that connect the peripheral and spinal nerves with the brain. The peripheral nerves are attached to the spinal cord by 31 pairs of spinal nerves.

A cross-section of the spinal cord reveals gray matter in the form of an H or butterfly surrounded on all sides by white matter. As in the cerebral hemispheres, the gray matter is composed mostly of cell bodies, whereas the white is made up of the myelinated axon fibers (Figure 8). The upper limbs of the gray matter are the *dorsal* or *posterior horns,* and the lower are the *ventral* or *anterior horns.* The white matter is grouped into dorsal, ventral, and lateral *columns* (Figure 8).

After reading this chapter, some individuals may prefer to skip to Chapters 20–22 on the meninges, blood supply, and ventricular system before proceeding to the chapters on the various pathways.

CLINICAL ASPECTS

A question that's frequently asked is: "Is there any relationship between brain size and intelligence?" The answer is no. The normal human brain has a volume ranging between 1,000–1,400 cm^3, and despite many studies no correlation has ever been found between great intelligence and a large brain. Individuals who have brains less than 1,000 cm^3 are most often mentally defective, although not all mental defectives have small brains.

In Alzheimer's disease, a chronic, progressive degenerative disease of the cerebral cortex that affects older people, there is frequently a widening of the sulci, which can be seen on a CT scan and used as a physical basis for confirming the diagnosis.

Chapter 3

Pain and Temperature Pathway from the Extremities and Trunk

Most people who consult a doctor do so because they are in pain. Therefore, a fundamental understanding of the pain and temperature pathway is essential for quick and accurate diagnosis. Fortunately, this is a simple pathway, and a good grasp of it is easily obtained.

The receptors of pain and temperature are found in the dermis and epidermis of the skin. Nerve fibers pass from the dermis toward the spinal cord, with the cell bodies being situated in the dorsal root ganglion (Figure 1). The fibers then enter the cord through the dorsal root of the spinal nerve and end in the dorsal horn of the gray matter. Here the first neuron synapses with a second one that then crosses to the contralateral (opposite) side of the cord in the ventral white commissure, enters the lateral white column, and ascends to the ventral posterolateral nucleus of the thalamus (Figure 1; see also Appendix III, Figure 3). This ascending bundle of crossed pain and temperature fibers is known as the *lateral spinothalamic tract*. In the ventral posterolateral (VPL) nucleus the axons of the lateral spinothalamic tract synapse with tertiary neurons that leave the thalamus and ascend in the internal capsule to reach the *postcentral gyrus* (Figure 1). The cortical gray matter of the postcentral gyrus (also known as area 3,1,2) is the primary somatic sensory area of the brain and is concerned with interpreting pain and temperature sensations, as well as other cutaneous sensations, such as pressure and touch (see following chapters).

ACCESSORY DETAILS

The primary pain and temperature axons have branches that synapse in the dorsal horn with short neurons that pass down to the ventral horn (Figure 1). Here these short *internuncial* (messenger) neurons synapse with motor neurons, the axons of which pass out through the ventral root and go out to voluntary muscles, causing movement. This involuntary motor response to a sensory stimulus is called a *reflex*. It is a defense mechanism of the nervous system that permits quick, automatic responses to painful and potentially damaging situations. The internuncials may cross over to the other side of the cord and stimulate motor neurons there, or they may descend or ascend the cord and stimulate motor neurons at different levels of the cord. It all depends on which group of muscles needs to be "called into action."

One interesting reflex involves the pupils of the eye, which dilate during severe pain. Thus, even though the patient may deny or not express his or her pain, the pupils will reveal it to the astute observer.

The dorsal root of the spinal nerve is composed of sensory (afferent) axons whose cell bodies are situated in the dorsal root ganglion. The ventral root, on the other hand, is made up of motor or efferent axons, the cell bodies of which are located in the gray matter of the ventral horn. In some cases the ventral root also has autonomic motor fibers (see Chapter 12).

The fibers of each dorsal root come from a fairly circumscribed area of skin known as a *dermatome*. There is, however, at each boundary of the dermatome an area that is supplied by the adjacent segmental nerves. This overlap acts as a kind of biologic "insurance." For example, if the second thoracic nerve (T_2) is severed, then many of the pain and temperature sensations from the skin area supplied by T_2 will be carried by the T_1 and T_3 sensory neurons (Figure 2). There is also an overlap pattern in the spinal cord. The entering axon, before it passes into the dorsal horn, sends branches that ascend and descend one spinal segment in the dorsolateral fasciculus (or column) of Lissauer and then enter the dorsal horn at that segment (Figure 2).

HISTORICAL ASPECTS

General anesthesia wasn't discovered until the period 1842–1846 by four Americans—Drs. Long, Jackson, Morton, and Wells—each working independently of the other. Before the use of ether, the patient would be given some alcohol to drink and then would be held on the table by strong men while the doctor operated. Speed was essential, and some doctors were able to do a complete amputation of the leg above the knee in 90 seconds.

Acupuncture has been used in China for thousands of years, but the exact way it works is still unknown. It is now believed that insertion of the

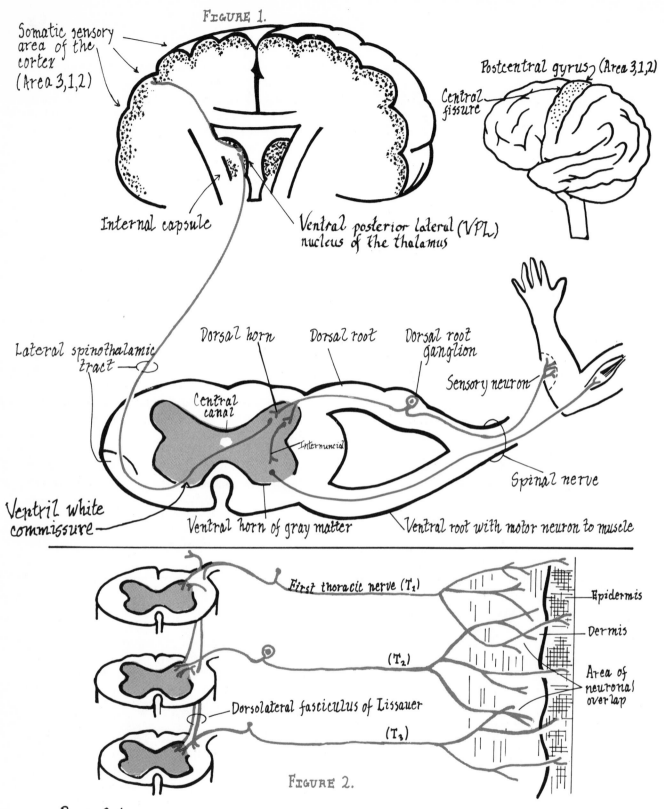

FIGURE 1.

Somatic sensory area of the cortex (Area 3,1,2)

Postcentral gyrus (Area 3,1,2)

Central fissure

Internal capsule

Ventral posterior lateral (VPL) nucleus of the thalamus

Dorsal horn

Dorsal root

Dorsal root ganglion

Sensory neuron

Lateral spinothalamic tract

Central canal

Intermuncial

Spinal nerve

Ventral white commissure

Ventral horn of gray matter

Ventral root with motor neuron to muscle

First thoracic nerve (T₁)

Epidermis

Dermis

(T₂)

Area of neuronal overlap

Dorsolateral fasciculus of Lissauer

(T₃)

FIGURE 2.

PLATE 3~1.

10

needles stimulates the body to release endorphins, which are morphine-like substances. In addition there is a great deal of suggestibility and autosuggestibility involved in its use. It must be stressed that acupuncture isn't a cure for the underlying cause of pain, but is an analgesic method that has best results with pain that involves the musculoskeletal system.

CLINICAL ASPECTS

The suffix -algia means pain; hence, neuralgia is pain in the nerves. An analgesic is some substance, such as morphine, aspirin, or alcohol, that deadens or dulls pain. (In the "Special Neuroanatomic and Neuropharmacologic Glossary" in Appendix I you will find interesting facts on various pharmacologic agents.) The suffix -esthesia, on the other hand, means sensations. Thus, an anesthetic is something that deadens or dulls all sensations.

A common cause of neuralgia is pressure from an intervertebral disc (a "slipped" disc in layperson's language) upon the spinal cord (Appendix IV, Figure 6) or spinal nerve that can produce great pain. If the condition occurs in the lumbar (lower back) area the pain most often radiates down the length of one leg, producing a condition known as sciatica.

Referred Pain

The pain pathway from the viscera (internal organs) is poorly understood. Visceral pain is not well localized; in certain cases it isn't felt at the organ site, but is experienced at the surface of the body some distance from the affected organ. Such a reaction is known as referred pain, and in many instances it is quite specific and can serve as an excellent diagnostic aid. For example, a person suffering from a coronary attack often experiences a sharp pain that radiates along the inner aspect of the left arm; pain originating from the ureters is felt in the inguinal area; pain from the lungs and diaphragm is experienced at the shoulders near the root of the neck.

Phantom Limb

In many cases following amputation the patient complains of excruciating pain from the fingers or toes that no longer exist! The explanation for this strange phenomenon is as follows. A stimulus applied anywhere along the nerve fiber is experienced by the sensory cortex as coming not from the site of stimulation, but rather from the skin area supplied by the nerves being stimulated. The nerve fibers at the stump are frequently squeezed by the scar tissue, and this pain stimulus passes to the sensory cortex, which interprets it as coming not from the stump area but from the skin areas of the fingers or toes of the missing limb.

Cordotomy

In cases of severe pain, as for example, from cancers or phantom limb, in which drugs no longer alleviate the pain, a surgical procedure known as *cordotomy* may be performed. The surgeon cuts the lateral spinothalamic tract of the cord on the opposite side from the site of the pain and at a level one or two segments higher than the entrance of the uppermost spinal nerve that serves the affected area. The latter is done because of the overlap that exists in the cord (see above). In some cases the cordotomy is done on both sides.

Syringomyelia

This is a rare degenerative disease of the spinal cord that begins in the central canal area of the cervical cord. As it expands it first destroys the adjacent ventral white commissure, producing the classical symptoms of loss of pain and temperature sensations only, in both upper limbs (Appendix IV, Figure 7).

DIAGNOSTIC TESTS

Pain

Have the patient close his or her eyes. With a pin, lightly prick the areas where pain sensations are thought to be absent. Ask when the patient feels the pin and when not.

Temperature

Take two test tubes, one with warm water and the other with cold. Again ask the patient to close the eyes. Alternately touch the test tubes to the areas where the sensations are believed to be lost and inquire whether the patient can feel the hot or cold.

Chapter 4

Pathway for Pressure and Simple (Crude) Touch from the Extremities and Trunk

The receptors for pressure and crude touch are situated in the dermis of the skin. The nerve fibers travel in the peripheral nerves toward the spinal cord. The cell bodies are aggregated in the dorsal root ganglion, and from here axons enter the cord through the dorsal root (Figure 1). Upon entering, the axons pass into the ipsilateral (i.e., the same side) dorsal white column and bifurcate. One branch immediately enters the dorsal horn gray matter and synapses with a second (or secondary) neuron. The other branch ascends in the ipsilateral dorsal column for as many as 10 spinal segments and then enters the dorsal horn gray matter to synapse with a second neuron (Figure 1). In both cases, the secondary neurons decussate (i.e., cross over to the other side) and enter the ventral white column, where they form the ventral spinothalamic tract. This tract ascends to the ventral posterolateral nucleus of the thalamus, where it synapses with third (or tertiary) neurons (Figure 1), which then relay the pressure and crude touch sensations to the postcentral gyrus of the cortex, which is concerned with interpreting sensations.

Many neuroanatomists claim and some books state that there is no basis for separating the lateral and ventral spinothalamic tracts and that the two are really one large bundle—the spinothalamic tract that has intermingled in it both pain and temperature axons, as well as those for pressure and simple touch.

These tracts may form one bundle but clinical data have shown that the pain and temperature fibers are concentrated in its lateral portion (i.e., in the lateral white columns), whereas the pressure and simple touch axons are situated in its ventral medial part (i.e., in the ventral white columns). So you can either say it's one bundle with a lateral and ventral portion or two adjacent bundles—the lateral and ventral spinothalamic tracts (and such are the controversies that divide neuroanatomists).

CLINICAL ASPECTS

Because one branch of the first neuron synapses immediately with a second neuron, whereas the second branch ascends ipsilaterally for many segments, injuries to the spinal cord rarely result in complete loss of pressure and crude touch sensations. For example, if there is any injury to the spinal cord at point A in Figure 1 and the ventral spinothalamic tract is cut, one sees that the long ascending branch of the primary neuron bypasses the injury (on the uninjured side), and thus the sensations can still reach the postcentral gyrus. Naturally, if the sensory cortex, the internal capsule, or the thalamus is injured, then the pressure and crude touch sensations are lost on the contralateral side of the body.

DIAGNOSTIC TEST FOR SIMPLE TOUCH

Have the patient close his or her eyes. Then gently stroke the skin area with a wisp of cotton and ask whether the patient feels it or not.

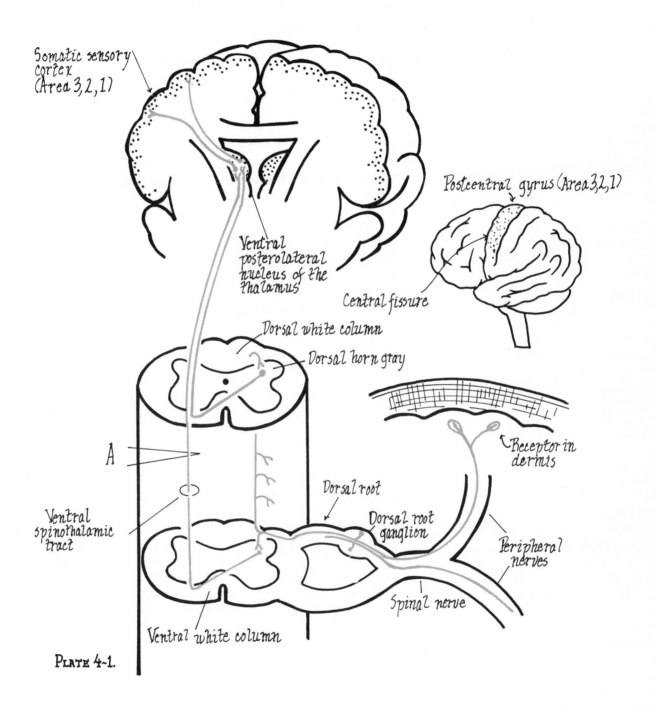

Somatic sensory cortex (Area 3,2,1)

Postcentral gyrus (Area 3,2,1)

Central fissure

Ventral posterolateral nucleus of the thalamus

Dorsal white column

Dorsal horn gray

A

Receptor in dermis

Dorsal root

Dorsal root ganglion

Ventral spinothalamic tract

Peripheral nerves

Spinal nerve

Ventral white column

PLATE 4-1.

13

Pathway for Proprioception, Fine (Discriminatory) Touch, and Vibratory Sense from the Extremities and Trunk

Three different sensations—proprioception, fine touch, and vibratory senses—all use the same pathway. *Proprioception* is the sense that enables one to know exactly and at all times where the parts of the body are in space and in relation to each other. Thus, it enables a person, with the eyes closed, to bring up the hand and touch the tip of the nose with the index finger. Its receptors are located in muscles, tendons, and joints. *Fine touch* is the sense that enables a person, again with the eyes closed, to identify various objects, such as keys, velvet, coins, and ping-pong balls, by touch. This property is known in medicine as *stereognosis*. Fine touch also involves the facility to discriminate between two points when being touched by both points simultaneously, as with the two points of a compass. These receptors are situated in the dermis of the skin, and they are most sensitive in the fingertips and lips and least sensitive on the back. *Vibratory sense* is, as its name implies, the sensation of vibrating objects.

The fibers of all three sensations pass toward the spinal cord in the peripheral nerves, and the cell bodies are aggregated in the dorsal root ganglion. From here, axons enter the spinal cord and immediately pass into the ipsilateral dorsal white columns, where they ascend all the way up to the medulla (Figure 1). Axons that enter the cord at the sacral and lumbar levels are situated in the medial part of the dorsal column, which is called the *fasciculus gracilis*, whereas those axons that enter at the thoracic and cervical levels form the more lateral *fasciculus cuneatus* (Figure 1). The axons of each fasciculus terminate in their respective nucleus in the medulla. The second-order neurons leave the nucleus gracilis and the nucleus cuneatus and cross over to the other side of the medulla, where they form a bundle known as the *medial lemniscus*, which ascends to the ventral posterolateral (VPL) nucleus of the thalamus (Figure 1). Here the second-order neurons synapse with third-order neurons that pass up through the internal capsule to reach the postcentral gyrus (area 3,1,2), which is the primary cerebral somesthetic (somatic sensory) region (Figure 2).

CLINICAL ASPECTS

Damage to the postcentral gyrus, to the medial lemniscus, to the dorsal column, or to the cell bodies in the dorsal root ganglion results in several distinct clinical symptoms:

1. Astereognosis, or loss of ability to distinguish between objects through touch and manipulation.
2. Loss of the vibratory sense.
3. Loss of two-point tactile discrimination—when touched simultaneously with two points of a compass, the patient reports feeling only one.
4. A loss of proprioception, so that there is an inability to know where the limbs are. Therefore, such a patient looks down at the feet when walking, and at night would stagger or fall. When asked to stand erect with both feet together and eyes closed, the patient's body sways—a positive Romberg sign.

If the injury is bilateral, then, of course, the symptoms will be on both sides of the body. If, however, the lesion is on one side, then the symptoms will appear on one side only, depending on where the damage is. If the damage is before the decussation—that is, in the dorsal root ganglion, the posterior column, or medullary nuclei—then the signs will be on the same side; if it is after the decussation—in the medial lemniscus, the thalamus, or cerebral cortex—then the signs will be on the side opposite the lesion.

Damage to the dorsal root ganglion frequently occurs in the third stage of syphilis when the bacterial organisms selectively attack and destroy the proprioceptive cell bodies, but initially spare those of pain, temperature, crude touch, and pressure. Tabetics (those who have the third stage of the dis-

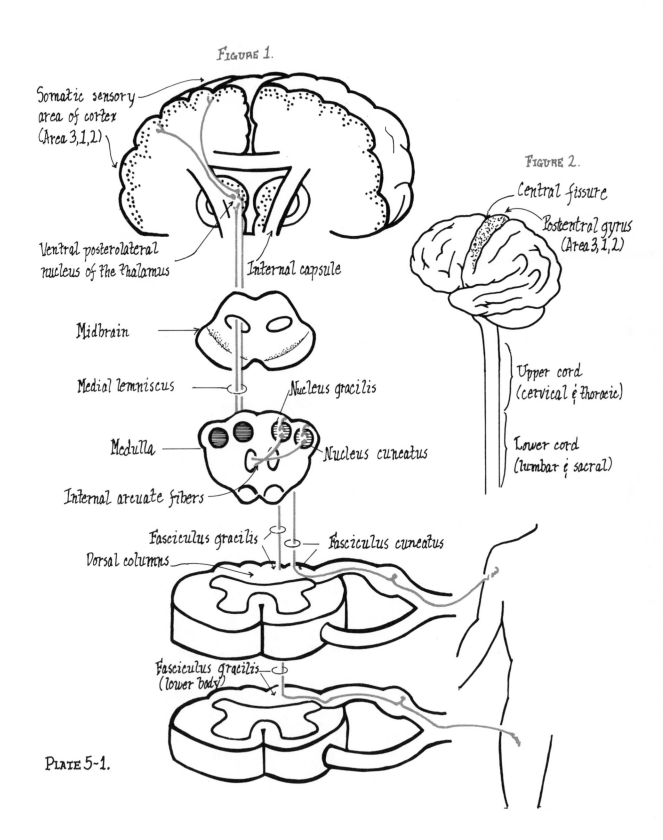

FIGURE 1.

Somatic sensory area of cortex (Area 3,1,2)

Ventral posterolateral nucleus of the thalamus

Internal capsule

Midbrain

Medial lemniscus

Nucleus gracilis

Medulla

Nucleus cuneatus

Internal arcuate fibers

Fasciculus gracilis

Fasciculus cuneatus

Dorsal columns

Fasciculus gracilis (lower body)

FIGURE 2.

Central fissure

Postcentral gyrus (Area 3,1,2)

Upper cord (cervical & thoracic)

Lower cord (lumbar & sacral)

PLATE 5-1.

15

ease) therefore exhibit *ataxia*, a characteristic staggering and lack of coordination.

DIAGNOSTIC TESTS

Have the patient close his or her eyes. Then place in succession different objects (e.g., a key, a coin, a matchbox) in the patient's hand and have the patient describe the shape, size, and consistency of the object and identify it.

With the patient's eyes still closed, ask him or her to touch the tip of the nose with the index finger, or have the patient stand erect and observe whether the patient sways when the eyes are closed. Failure to perform either task indicates proprioceptive impairment.

HISTORICAL NOTE

Syphilis has been present in the New World for thousands of years, but it only appeared in Europe in 1495 at the siege of Naples. From there it spread rapidly throughout the Continent and became one of the most feared and prevalent diseases. The French called it the Italian disease, the Italians in turn called it the Spanish disease, the Spaniards called it the English disease, and so on. Therapy then consisted of spreading a cream containing mercury over the affected area for a period of several months. This gave rise to the joke that "you spend one night with Venus and six months with Mercury."* This scourge was finally cured with the discovery of Salvarsan by Paul Erlich. Salvarsan was also known as "606" because 606 experiments were done until he discovered it. Today penicillin is the drug of choice in the treatment of this illness.

---

*Mercury in those days was called "quacksalver," which later became "quicksilver," a word that is still used today. From "quacksalver" came the word "quack" or one who prescribes quacksalver (the treatment really didn't help very much).

Chapter 6

Sensory Pathways from the Face and Related Areas

Our discussions of somatic sensory pathways have so far not included descriptions of nerves from the face and related areas because these areas do not "use" the spinal nerves. Sensations for these areas pass in the fifth cranial nerve, the trigeminal. The basic groundplan is pretty much the same, and an understanding of it is important, especially for those studying dentistry or who have chosen a specialty involving the cranial region.

The trigeminal nerve is the major somatic sensory nerve for the face, the anterior half of the scalp, the mouth cavity, the meninges, the sinuses, the teeth, the tongue, the cornea and rest of the eyeball, and the outer surface of the eardrum. It transmits the sensations of pain and temperature and all kinds of touch, pressure, and proprioception, but not those of the special senses, such as hearing, taste, smell, vision, and equilibrium, which are carried by other cranial nerves.

PAIN AND TEMPERATURE PATHWAY

The pain and temperature pathway for the face and its adjacent regions is shown by the solid lines in Figure 1. From receptors situated in the above-mentioned areas, fibers pass in the peripheral branches of the trigeminal nerve toward the brain. Their cell bodies are located in the *semilunar* or *Gasserian ganglion* (Figure 1), which is the analogue of the dorsal root ganglion. From here the axons enter the pons and are immediately concentrated in a bundle, the descending or spinal tract of cranial nerve V, which swings down and in many cases reaches the upper cervical region of the cord. Along this course the primary neurons peel off and enter the adjacent nucleus of the descending tract of cranial nerve V, where they synapse with secondary neurons. These leave the nucleus, cross over to the contralateral side, and ascend to terminate in the ventral posteromedial (VPM) nucleus of the thalamus (Figure 1). This crossed pain and temperature bundle is called the ventral secondary ascending tract of cranial nerve V (or the ventral trigeminal tract) and is analogous to the lateral spinothalamic tract. From the thalamus, tertiary neurons pass into the internal capsule, ascend in it, and end in the postcentral gyrus (area 3,1,2)—the primary or main somesthetic region of the cortex.

PRESSURE AND TOUCH PATHWAY

These neurons (represented by the dashed lines in Figure 1) also have their cell bodies in the semilunar ganglion, but their axons terminate immediately in the main sensory nucleus of cranial nerve V, situated in the pons (Figure 1). The secondary neurons reach the ventral posteromedial nucleus of the thalamus via the dorsal secondary ascending tract of cranial nerve V (or the dorsal trigeminal tract) which is a crossed and uncrossed tract. That is, some axons travel ipsilaterally and some contralaterally. Tertiary neurons are relayed from the thalamus to the postcentral gyrus (Figure 1). Thus we see that, whereas pain and temperature are projected on the contralateral cerebral cortex, pressure and touch are bilaterally projected. Therefore, if one side of the sensory cortex is damaged, the patient will suffer no loss of pressure or touch from the face, but will lose the pain and temperature feelings on the contralateral side.

PROPRIOCEPTION PATHWAY

This pathway is composed of trigemino-proprioceptive fibers from the muscles of mastication, the temporomandibular joint, and the peridontal ligament around the teeth. However, the trigemino-proprioceptive fibers are an exception in that their primary cell bodies aren't in a ganglion outside the CNS, but are situated in the mesencephalic nucleus in the midbrain (Figure 2). The further pathway of this sensation to the postcentral gyrus is not well known.

ACCESSORY DETAIL

There are several reflexes involving the trigeminal nerve, of which the most important is the corneal or "blink" reflex. If an object touches the cornea of one eye, both eyes will blink immediately. The pathway is as follows: the touch stimulus from the cornea reaches the ipsilateral main sensory nucleus of

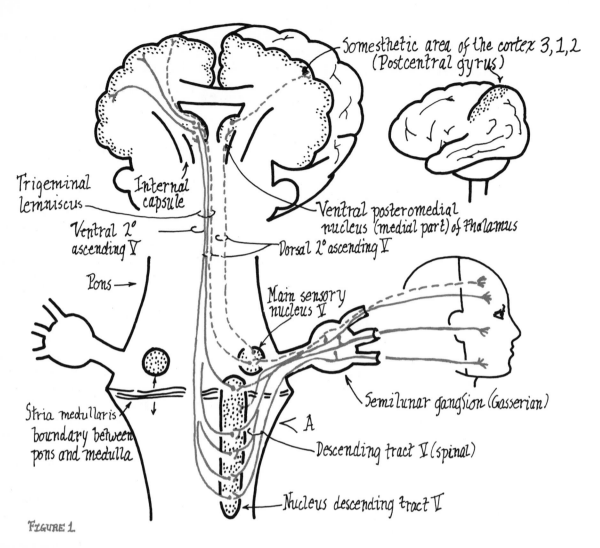

Somesthetic area of the cortex 3,1,2 (Postcentral gyrus)

Trigeminal lemniscus

Internal capsule

Ventral posteromedial nucleus (medial part) of Thalamus

Ventral 2° ascending Ⅴ

Dorsal 2° ascending Ⅴ

Pons →

Main sensory nucleus Ⅴ

Semilunar ganglion (Gasserian)

Stria medullaris boundary between pons and medulla

< A

Descending tract Ⅴ (spinal)

Nucleus descending tract Ⅴ

FIGURE 1.

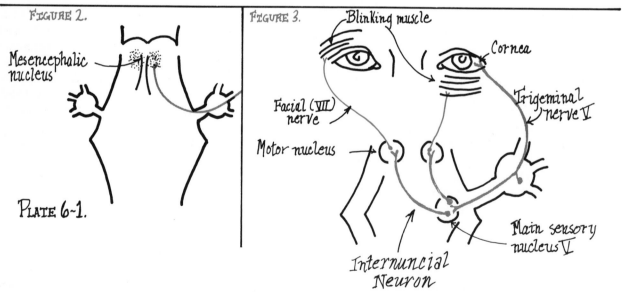

FIGURE 2.

Mesencephalic nucleus

PLATE 6-1.

FIGURE 3.

Blinking muscle

Cornea

Facial (Ⅶ) nerve

Trigeminal nerve Ⅴ

Motor nucleus

Internuncial Neuron

Main sensory nucleus Ⅴ

cranial nerve V. This sends out internuncial neurons that pass to the *right and left* motor nuclei of the facial nerve. From here motor neurons pass out and stimulate the muscles that cause blinking (Figure 3).

CLINICAL ASPECTS

Reflexes not only are a defense mechanism, but also are useful diagnostically, enabling the physician to test the integrity of nerve pathways. If, upon testing, a reflex is not elicited, the physician then has to find out where the interruption in the pathway is: in the sensory pathway, the internuncial connections, or the motor pathway. In addition, there are reflexes that appear only in pathologic conditions, informing the physician that something is wrong.

When a person is anesthetized in surgery, specific reflexes disappear as deeper and deeper levels of unconsciousness are reached. Thus, the anesthetist is able to gauge accurately the level of unconsciousness by means of the presence or absence of these reflexes.

If the trigeminal nerve is transected or the semilunar ganglion is damaged, then the individual will suffer loss of all facial sensations on the same side as the injury. As mentioned previously, injury to one side of the sensory cortex, internal capsule, etc. results in loss of facial pain and temperature sensation contralaterally, but pressure and touch remain.

Trigeminal neuralgia (tic douloureux) is a condition of unknown etiology in which the patient suffers excruciating, shooting pain on one side of the face. Because drugs don't often bring relief, surgical treatment is used. The descending tract of cranial nerve V lies superficially, thus enabling neurosurgeons to go in and cut it on the side that has the pain (point A in Figure 1). Thus they sever the pain and temperature axons while sparing the pressure and touch fibers.

Brain tissue itself has no sensations whatsoever, and therefore operations on it can be done using only local anesthetics. Headaches are usually the result of pressure or pain in nonnervous structures on or within the brain or skull, such as the arteries or the meninges (the coverings of the brain). They can be caused by many factors, and there are many types of headaches. Among the most common are migraine, cluster, and tension headaches.

The exact cause of migraine is unknown, but it tends to run in families and to affect women three times as much as men. The individual generally has one or two attacks per month that each last from several hours to a couple of days. The attack is generally preceded by a visual aura, such as "stars in front of the eyes," and then there is a severe throbbing pain on one side of the head that is often accompanied by nausea and vomiting. The pain is due to severe dilation of cerebral arteries on one side of the head.* Migraine headaches are treated by taking drugs of the ergotamine family that produce vasoconstriction, thereby preventing the dilation and pain.

Cluster headaches are sudden, severe, often retrobulbar headaches that occur once a day over a period of 2–3 months. The cause is unknown, but they are ten times more frequent in men than women, occur most often at night, and are frequently triggered by drinking alcoholic drinks.

In tension headache, which is probably the most common and widespread type, there is a dull, steady ache often encircling the head like a hatband. It's believed that the many and varied stresses of modern life, along with fatigue and bottled up anger, cause the muscles of the head and neck to tense up and by doing so constrict nerves and arteries, which in turn produces the headaches. These can be relieved by ingesting aspirin and similar drugs, taking hot baths to relax the muscles and mind, and by massaging the scalp, neck, and shoulders to reduce muscular tension.

Tumors can also produce headaches due to increased intracranial pressure, but here the headaches are often accompanied by a projectile-type of vomiting.

---

*See Appendix VI, "Odds and Ends," for the interesting derivation of the word "migraine."

Chapter 7

Pathway for
Voluntary Muscle Activity

Everyone has undoubtedly seen at one time or another individuals who can't walk and are confined to wheelchairs, or who walk slowly, dragging one leg, or whose arm lies helplessly flexed on one side; in short, persons who have some form of paralysis. In most of these conditions the muscles are fundamentally intact, and the condition is due to some kind of injury to the nerves. Because damage to no other pathway is responsible for so much suffering and sorrow, a first-class understanding of this pathway is mandatory.

The *corticospinal tract* is the main tract for nearly all voluntary muscle activity. It originates in the precentral gyrus (area 4, the motor cortex) of the frontal lobe. Here are located its large cell bodies. Because many of these have a pyramidal shape, the corticospinal tract is also called the *pyramidal tract.** (How a conscious wish is "translated" into cortical nerve impulses is an age-old question involving the mind-matter problem and probably will never be answered satisfactorily.) From the cell bodies, axons leave the cortex and pass down through the internal capsule, which isn't a capsule but is rather the main passageway for ascending and descending fiber tracts (Figure 1). Leaving the internal capsule, the axon fibers pass down into the basis pedunculi of the midbrain and continue down the brainstem to reach the medulla oblongata. Here about 80–90% of the axons decussate to the opposite or contralateral side of the medulla and, having crossed over, descend in the spinal cord (Figure 1). Because these descending fibers are situated in the lateral white columns of the cord they are called the *lateral corticospinal tract*. Those axons that do not cross over in the medulla continue down on the same side to enter the ventral white columns of the spinal cord and are therefore known as the *ventral corticospinal tract*.

At each level of the cord, axons from the lateral corticospinal tract peel off and enter the gray matter of the ventral horn, where they terminate by synapsing with second-order neurons. At each corresponding level of the cord, axons of the ventral corticospinal tract peel off and cross over to the

other side of the cord (Figure 1). Here they also enter and terminate upon second-order neurons in the ventral horn. It must be emphasized that, in their entire course from the precentral gyrus to the ventral horn, both the lateral and ventral corticospinal tracts consist of single uninterrupted neurons; that is, the tracts are a single neuron pathway. These neurons are called *upper motor neurons*. The second-order neurons on which the upper motor neurons synapse send their axons out of the spinal cord via the ventral roots. They then branch out in the peripheral nerves and supply the voluntary muscles. These second-order neurons are *lower motor neurons*, and this differentiation between them and the upper motor neurons is very important clinically, as we shall soon see. In a person who is 6 feet tall, the axons that supply the toe muscles are nearly a yard long. The upper motor neurons begin in the precentral gyrus and end in the lower part of the cord, whereas the lower motor neuron begins in the lower cord and its axon passes down to supply the muscle situated on the sole of the foot.

DETAILS

Cerebral Localization

The nerve cell bodies of the upper motor neurons are arranged in a specific pattern in the gray matter of the precentral gyrus, so that neurons supplying the foot and leg muscles are situated dorsomedially in the gyrus. As one passes inferolaterally one finds the areas for the abdomen, chest, arm, hand, and face. One can describe this more colorfully by saying that the pattern is that of a person hanging upside down, with the feet in the longitudinal fissure and the head at the edge of the lateral fissure (Figure 1). The area of neurons that supplies the muscles of the hand is disproportionately large, reflecting the great number of neurons needed to carry out such fine and complicated movements as violin playing, surgery, and writing. This localization is also seen in the internal capsule, the main cerebral passageway for ascending and descending fiber tracts. In a horizontal section (Figure 1a) of the cerebral hemisphere one sees that the internal capsule consists of an anterior limb, a posterior limb,

*Others say that it is called the pyramidal tract because it decussates in the pyramids of the medulla.

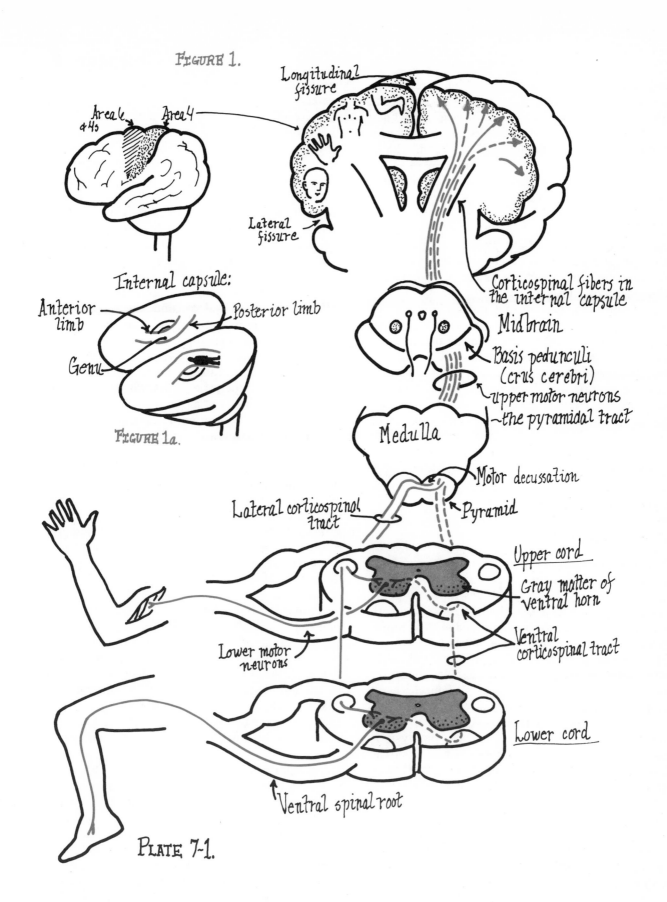

FIGURE 1.

Longitudinal fissure

Area 6 & 45   Area 4

Lateral fissure

Corticospinal fibers in the internal capsule

Internal capsule:

Anterior limb   Posterior limb

Genu

FIGURE 1a.

Midbrain

Basis pedunculi (crus cerebri)

upper motor neurons ~ the pyramidal tract

Medulla

Motor decussation

Lateral corticospinal tract

Pyramid

Upper cord

Gray matter of ventral horn

Ventral corticospinal tract

Lower motor neurons

Lower cord

Ventral spinal root

PLATE 7-1.

21

and a connecting area between them, called the *genu*. The fibers that supply the face are situated in the genu, and those supplying the rest of the body are found in the anterior two-thirds of the posterior limb. If the genu is damaged, then the muscles of the face are affected, but if the middle part of the posterior limb is injured, then the leg muscles will not receive nervous supply.

Suppressor Part of the Pyramidal Tract

Not all the neurons of the pyramidal tract have their origins in the precentral gyrus. Many of them originate in areas 4s and 6, which lie just anterior to the precentral gyrus (Figure 1). Pyramidal tract fibers originating here do not initiate impulses to voluntary muscles, but act as inhibitors, suppressors, or "brakes" on the lower motor neurons and prevent them from overdischarging when responding reflexively to sensory stimuli. If for some reason the suppressor fibers are damaged, then the lower motor neurons are freed from their control and fire excessively in response to reflex stimuli or discharge spontaneously. These conditions are known as *hyperreflexion* and *spasticity*, respectively, and are discussed in the text section.

CLINICAL ASPECTS

Lower Motor Neuron Paralysis

The best examples of lower motor neuron paralysis are when a nerve to a muscle is cut or when the cell bodies of the ventral horn are destroyed by poliomyelitis virus, which selectively attacks them. In both cases the muscles are deprived of their immediate nerve supply; they are unable to contract and become soft, flabby, and atrophic—characteristics of a flaccid paralysis. Naturally, because the motor limb of the reflex arc is damaged, the muscles can't respond reflexively to sensory stimuli.

If the cell bodies are destroyed, as in polio, then the axons cannot regenerate and the paralysis is permanent. If, however, a nerve is cut, then the part of the axon attached to the cell body can regenerate, and some of the functions can be restored (see Chapter 1).

Upper Motor Neuron Paralysis

Upper motor neuron paralysis occurs when there is damage to the corticospinal tract anywhere along its path: the cell bodies in the precentral gyrus or their descending axons in the internal capsule, brainstem, or spinal cord. The most common site of injury is in the cerebral hemisphere, before the de-

cussation. Injury results most often when an artery becomes stopped up and the neurons, deprived of their oxygen supply, die, producing what is known as a cerebrovascular accident (CVA) or, in popular language, a *stroke*. If the site affected is above the motor decussation, then the signs and symptoms will be seen in the muscles on the opposite side of the body. If the injury is below the decussation—say, a cut in the left half of the spinal cord—then the ensuing paralysis will be on the same side as the damage. This type of paralysis is different from a lower motor neuron paralysis in a number of essential ways. First of all, the lower motor neurons are not affected and the reflex arc is complete, and thus reflexes can be elicited. Second, the suppressor fibers originating in areas 4s and 6 are knocked out, and their braking effect on the lower motor neurons is no longer effective. The lower motor neurons now overdischarge to stimuli or even fire spontaneously. Clinically, this hyperreflexia manifests itself as follows: when the wrist of a paralyzed arm is grasped firmly, there will be a series of rapid, strong, muscular contractions, known as *clonus*. When the lower motor neurons discharge spontaneously, the muscles contract strongly, a condition known as *spasticity*. This upper motor neuron paralysis is spastic, as opposed to lower motor neuron paralysis, which is flaccid. In upper motor neuron paralysis a characteristic and specific type of reflex—the *Babinski reflex*—can be elicited. When the sole of the foot of a healthy person is stroked in a heel-to-toe direction, the toes will curl. However, in a patient who has an upper motor neuron lesion, the toes will fan apart and the big toe will flex dorsally. The exact route and mechanism of the Babinski reflex are still not fully understood. (In a normal infant up to the age of 6 months or so, in whom the myelinization of the axons is not complete, a Babinski response can be elicited routinely.) Also, certain superficial reflexes, such as the abdominal and cremasteric, which are elicited when the skin is stroked, are lost. Once again the exact reason and mechanism are not clear.

A person who is "paralyzed" on one side of the body can frequently make crude movements of the trunk musculature on the affected side. The explanation for this is as follows: It is known that some of the lateral corticospinal fibers do not cross over at all, and it is believed that these uncrossed fibers, along with some of the crossed ones, supply the muscles of the trunk. Thus the trunk muscles of each side receive axons from both the right and left cerebral cortex. This arrangement is known as *bilateral innervation*.

Because a CVA may not destroy all the upper motor neuron axons to a group of muscles, those remaining intact can be utilized to regain some of the lost functions. This requires rehabilitation and involves such personnel as physiotherapists and occupational therapists.

Paralytic conditions may be defined according to the part(s) of the body affected: *monoplegia* is paralysis of either an upper or a lower limb; *hemiplegia* is paralysis of an upper and a lower limb on the same side; *paraplegia* is paralysis of both lower limbs; *quadriplegia* is paralysis of all four limbs.

Cerebral Palsy

Cerebral palsy (CP) is the name given to a large group of motor disorders of infants and children in which there is paralysis or disturbed motion (e.g., spasticity, tremors, athetosis, etc.) caused by brain damage. There may also be disturbed posture and muscle tone. In addition, mental retardation and other neurologic symptoms are often present. Damage to the brain may occur in utero, during delivery, or postpartum and may be due to infection or difficulties during delivery, such as trauma, decreased oxygen supply, etc. Other cases are idiopathic; that is, from unknown causes. Generally one sees gross or microscopic lesions in the precentral gyrus, the pyramidal tract, or in the extrapyramidal system, but in some cases there is no demonstrable brain pathology. The early detection of cerebral palsy is difficult because the corticospinal tracts aren't completely myelinated until the child is 1–1½ years of age.

Amyotrophic Lateral Sclerosis (ALS)—Lou Gehrig's Disease*

This is a chronic, progressive, degenerative disease that selectively attacks the corticospinal tracts in the lateral white columns. The disease generally begins at the midcord level and progresses upward, sparing sensations and intellect. As a result one sees the typical triad of muscle weakness, muscle wasting, and hyperreflexia in the hand, forearm, and later the shoulder girdle. Like so many other neurologic diseases there is no known cause, cure, or means of prevention for ALS, and it ends fatally within 3–5 years.

HISTORICAL NOTES

Hippocrates, one of the greatest physicians in history, noted over 2,000 years ago that injuries to one side of the head often produced paralysis on the contralateral (opposite) side of the body. Later Aretaeus of Cappadocia (circa 120–200 A.D.) said that this fact must be due to the nerves crossing somewhere in their pathway.

---

*Lou Gehrig was one of baseball's greatest players. Between 1925 and 1938 he played 2,310 consecutive games for the New York Yankees and was the Most Valuable Player in 1927, 1931, 1934, and 1936. He had a lifetime batting average of .350 and also batted in more than 100 runs/year in 13 years. In 1927, he hit .376 and along with Babe Ruth (.356), Early Combs (.356), and Tony Lazzer (.309) formed the batting sequence known as "Murderer's Row": one can imagine the nervous condition of the pitchers who had to face them. Lou Gehrig died in 1941 at the age of 38 from amyotrophic lateral sclerosis.

Chapter 8

Pathway to Voluntary Muscles
of the Head

Our discussion of the pyramidal tract centered on those fibers that descend into the spinal cord and synapse there with lower motor neurons that go out and innervate voluntary muscles of the body. It did not include fibers to the voluntary muscles of the head because the lower motor neurons supplying them are not situated in the spinal nerves but are associated with cranial nerves originating in the brainstem. The basic framework, however, is the same as for the corticospinal tracts. It is a two-neuron pathway consisting of an upper motor neuron originating in the cerebral cortex, the axon of which descends and synapses with a lower motor neuron, which in turn goes out and stimulates voluntary muscles.

The cell bodies of the upper motor neurons are located in the lowest part of the precentral gyrus (motor cortex—area 4) adjacent to the lateral fissure (Figure 1). There is in addition another motor area for eyeball movements, which is situated in the middle frontal gyri (Figure 1a). Axons from here join descending fibers from the face area, and together they pass through the genu of the internal capsule. Because the fibers then enter the brainstem, or bulb, and terminate on lower motor neurons, they are called the *corticobulbar tract* in contradistinction to the corticospinal tract. The cell bodies of the lower motor neurons are concentrated in specific areas of the brainstem called *nuclei*, and their axons form many of the cranial nerves. These nerves differ from spinal nerves in that the sensory and motor fibers do not separate into dorsal and ventral roots. Furthermore, some cranial nerves have no sensory axons; all their fibers are lower motor neurons. To complicate the matter even further, there are cranial nerves that are entirely sensory in their makeup. Be that as it may, the cranial nerves that interest us here are those whose axons supply voluntary muscles. These are the oculomotor (III) and the trochlear (IV) nerves, whose nuclei are situated in the midbrain and whose axons go out to supply five of the six eyeball muscles and the levator palpebrae superioris; the trigeminal (V), the abducens (VI), and the facial (VII) nerves, all of which originate in the pons. The trigeminal nerve innervates the muscles of mastication, as well as the anterior belly of the digastric, mylohyoid, tensor tympani, and tensor veli palatini muscles; the abducens supplies the last remaining eyeball muscle; the facial nerve, as its name implies, supplies all the muscles of facial expression. Finally, in the medulla are situated the nucleus of the glossopharyngeal nerve (IX), which innervates a single muscle in the pharynx (throat); the nucleus of the vagus nerve (X), which supplies muscles in the throat concerned with talking and swallowing (the nucleus of IX and X is really a single common nucleus called the *nucleus ambiguus*); the nucleus of the hypoglossal nerve (XII), which supplies all the muscles of the tongue; and the accessory nerve (XI), which is an exception in that it doesn't supply muscles in the head but rather two very important ones in the neck—the sternomastoid and the trapezius.

No mention has yet been made of the crossing over of the corticobulbar tract because it isn't the same for all the cranial nerves just mentioned. The motor nuclei of all the cranial nerves mentioned, except VII and XII, receive innervation from both the right and left corticobulbar tracts; that is, each corticobulbar tract supplies both the right and left cranial nuclei (Figure 1). This bilateral innervation is a kind of biologic insurance. If the right tract is damaged, for example, the nuclei will still receive the upper motor neuron impulses from the intact left corticobulbar tract and there will be no impairment of muscle function.

The nuclei of cranial nerve XII, the hypoglossal nerve, receive only contralateral innervation; that is, the nucleus of the right side is supplied by axons from the left corticobulbar tract and vice versa. The clinical implication is fairly obvious: a lesion to the left corticobulbar tract would result in loss of nerve supply to the right nucleus, and the muscles of the right side of the tongue would be paralyzed.

The facial nucleus, cranial nerve VII, combines features of both types of nuclei discussed so far. Its nucleus is divided into an upper part, which supplies the muscles of the upper half of the face, and a lower part, which supplies muscles in the lower half. The upper part of the nucleus receives bilateral innervation from the corticobulbar tract, whereas the lower part receives its supply from the contralateral tract (Figure 2).

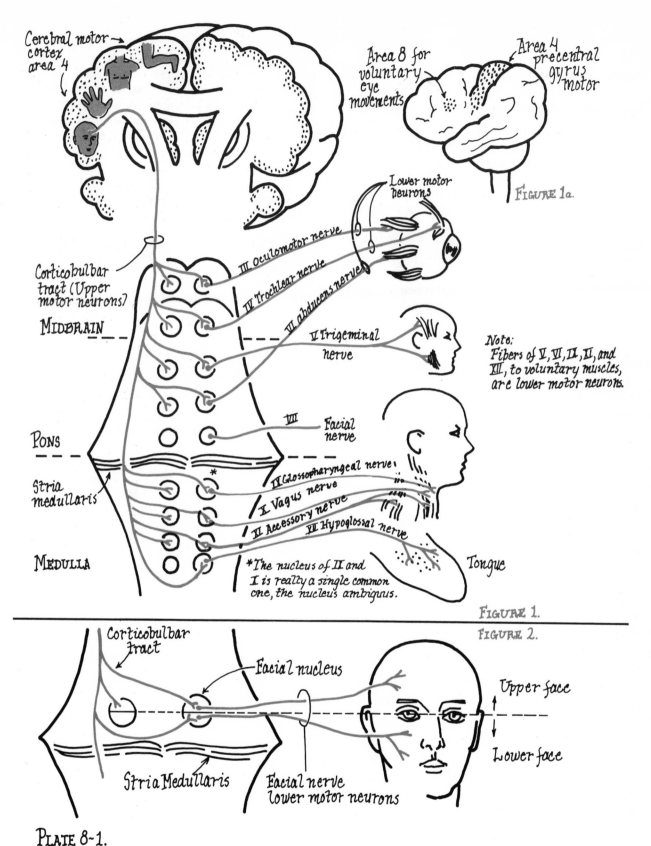

Cerebral motor cortex area 4

Area 8 for voluntary eye movements

Area 4 precentral gyrus motor

FIGURE 1a.

Lower motor neurons

Corticobulbar tract (Upper motor neurons)

MIDBRAIN

III Oculomotor nerve

IV Trochlear nerve

VI abducens nerve

V Trigeminal nerve

Note:
Fibers of V, VI, IX, XI, and XII, to voluntary muscles, are lower motor neurons.

PONS

VII Facial nerve

Stria medullaris

IX Glossopharyngeal nerve

X Vagus nerve

XI Accessory nerve

XII Hypoglossal nerve

MEDULLA

*The nucleus of XI and X is really a single common one, the nucleus ambiguus.

Tongue

FIGURE 1.

FIGURE 2.

Corticobulbar tract

Facial nucleus

Upper face

Lower face

Stria Medullaris

Facial nerve lower motor neurons

PLATE 8-1.

CLINICAL ASPECTS

Upper Motor Neuron Lesion

As we have just seen, all the cranial motor nuclei (except the lower part of the facial and hypoglossal nerves) receive bilateral innervation. Therefore, if there is a lesion in one of the corticobulbar tracts, none of the nuclei or the muscles they supply would be affected. However, an upper motor neuron lesion (also known as a supranuclear lesion) could affect cranial nerve XII and/or the lower part of VII. If corticobulbar fibers to the facial nucleus are damaged, there is paralysis of the lower part of the facial muscles on the side opposite the lesion (Figure 2). The paralysis is spastic, and reflexes are present. Because the upper part of the facial muscles receives bilateral innervation, the patient can still move the brow on the paralyzed side of the face (Figure 2). If corticobulbar neurons to the hypoglossal nucleus are destroyed, the tongue muscles on the contralateral side will be paralyzed but will not atrophy (Figure 1). When the patient is asked to protrude the tongue, the muscles on the unaffected side cause it to deviate to the side on which the muscles are paralyzed.

Lower Motor Neuron Lesions

Lower motor neuron lesions are discussed in Chapter 13.

Chapter 9

Subcortical Motor Areas

In lower forms of animals, such as sharks and birds, which do not have a cerebral motor cortex, movement is initiated by a group of nuclei, the basal ganglia, together with other subcortical areas. Such movement is highly coordinated and often very quick, but it is instinctive and crude. In humans there has been added to this old motor system a new, "higher" one—the cerebral motor cortex—which enables us to perform exceptionally skilled and purposeful movements, especially with the hands. This new system is called the pyramidal system, whereas the older, cruder one is the extrapyramidal system. For a while it was thought that the two were independent of each other, but now it is known that they are interconnected. Our knowledge of the old system is very incomplete, and a lot of what we think today may have to be modified by new discoveries tomorrow. With respect to terminology, there has been a tendency recently to use terms other than pyramidal and extrapyramidal, but this change in semantics hasn't been accompanied by any great increase in understanding. Also, many of the nuclei are grouped together and given special names (e.g., corpus striatum, lentiform nuclei). Because different authors don't always mean the same thing by the same term, in this book the nuclei and areas will be named individually.

Deep in the cerebral hemispheres are three well-defined nuclei—the *caudate nucleus*, which lies medial to the anterior limb of the internal capsule, and the *globus pallidus* and *putamen*, which lie lateral to the genu (Figure 1; see also Appendix III, Figure 3). These three plus the amygdala constitute the basal ganglia. (The author has never been able to find out why the amygdala, which is concerned with olfactory reflexes, is considered a basal ganglion.) In the diencephalon is located the subthalamic nucleus of Luys, whereas in the midbrain are the red nucleus, the substantia nigra, and the reticular formation (Figure 2). All the above-mentioned structures make up the subcortical or primitive motor areas.

Various areas of the cerebral motor cortex, including areas 4, 4s, and 6, send fibers to the caudate, putamen, and pallidus (Figure 3). The globus pallidus, which also receives fibers from the caudate and putamen, is the main discharge center and is therefore connected with the subthalamic nucleus, substantia nigra, reticular formation, and red nucleus (Figure 3). In addition, the subthalamic nucleus and substantia nigra are connected to the reticular formation and red nucleus, which discharge to the lower motor neurons at all levels of the cord via the reticulospinal and rubrospinal tracts (Figure 3). Thus, there is, as was so aptly described by the neuroanatomist Elliot, a "cascading effect" with respect to nuclei and their discharges. Finally, the globus pallidus is connected to the thalamus by two tracts, the *ansa lenticularis* and the *lenticular fasciculus*. As they enter the thalamus these two tracts merge to form the *thalamic fasciculus*. The thalamus in turn is connected back to the caudate and areas 4, 4s, and 6, thus establishing a feedback mechanism. If our knowledge of the interconnections between different subcortical nuclei and their relationship to areas 4, 4s, and 6 is poor, then our understanding of how they operate and regulate motor activity is almost nil.

CLINICAL ASPECTS

Lesions in the primitive subcortical nuclei produce several diseases characterized by disturbances of muscle tone and various abnormal involuntary movements (dyskinesia). The most common and best known of these is *parkinsonism*, a slow, progressive, degenerative disease of older people first described by Dr. James Parkinson, a 19th-century English physician, which afflicts over half a million people in the United States. Clinically, one sees a great increase in muscle tonus, leading to rigidity and slowness of movement (bradykinesia). The face often loses all signs of expression and becomes mask-like due to this hypertonicity. Combined with this is tremor, seen especially in the arms and hands, where it manifests itself in a characteristic pill-rolling motion. This tremor is most evident when the patient isn't doing anything with the hands—a resting tremor—but often disappears during purposeful movements. During walking, the head and shoulders are stooped, the gait is short and shuffling, and there is a loss of automatic movements, such as swinging of the arms.

The cause of the disease is unknown—it strikes every ethnic, socioeconomic, and national group—but at autopsy one sees degeneration of the substantia nigra and globus pallidus. It has been shown that dopamine is an essential neurotrans-

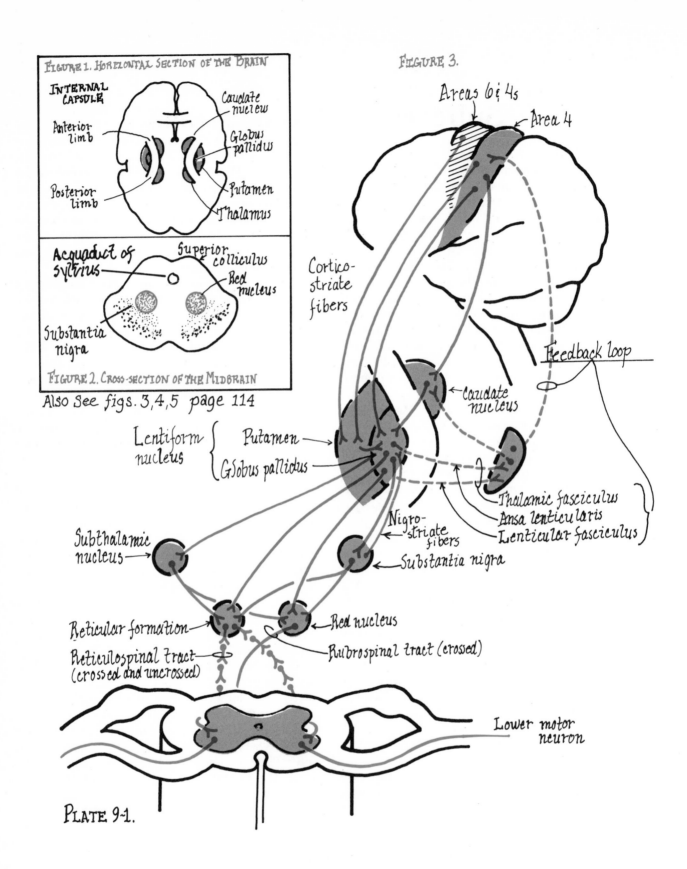

FIGURE 1. HORIZONTAL SECTION OF THE BRAIN

INTERNAL CAPSULE

Caudate nucleus

Anterior limb

Globus pallidus

Posterior limb

Putamen

Thalamus

Acquaduct of Sylvius

Superior colliculus

Red nucleus

Substantia nigra

FIGURE 2. CROSS-SECTION OF THE MIDBRAIN

Also See figs. 3,4,5 page 114

FIGURE 3.

Areas 6 & 4s

Area 4

Cortico-striate fibers

Feedback loop

Caudate nucleus

Lentiform nucleus { Putamen
Globus pallidus

Thalamic fasciculus
Ansa lenticularis
Lenticular fasciculus

Nigro-striate fibers

Subthalamic nucleus

Substantia nigra

Reticular formation

Red nucleus

Reticulospinal tract (crossed and uncrossed)

Rubrospinal tract (crossed)

Lower motor neuron

PLATE 9-1.

mitter in the basal ganglia. It is produced in the substantia nigra of the midbrain and passes up fibers to be used in the basal ganglia (Figure 3). In most cases of parkinsonism the substantia nigra is destroyed, and as a result there is a decrease in the amount of dopamine reaching the basal ganglia, thus producing the signs and symptoms of the illness. On the basis of this theory rests one of the current methods of treatment—that of supplying the basal ganglia with the missing dopamine. Dopamine cannot be given directly, however, because it does not pass the blood-brain barrier (see Chapter 1). Therefore, L-dopa, a necessary precursor of dopamine, is given because it can pass the blood-brain barrier and is then synthesized into dopamine. One often sees great improvement in patients following the administration of L-dopa, but as the disease progresses it has less of a beneficial effect and symptoms reappear along with the appearance of L-dopa side effects.

New developments have recently taken place in parkinsonism research.* Several young drug addicts developed very rapidly parkinsonian-like disease, and one who died revealed at autopsy destruction of the substantia nigra. Investigating further, researchers found that the addicts had used synthetic narcotics that had become contaminated with MPTP (N-methyl-4 phenyl 1,2,5,6 tetrahydropyridine) that brought on the parkinsonian-like condition. MPTP can also cause irreversible

parkinsonism in monkeys by destroying their substantia nigra. So at last this condition can be reproduced experimentally in animals, but the question still remains: what causes parkinsonism in older people? Parkinsonian-like symptoms may be seen in other conditions, such as Wilson's disease, in which there is abnormal copper metabolism that results in copper deposition in the globus pallidus, putamen, and liver, causing their degeneration. In mental patients high doses of chlorpromazine often produce signs of parkinsonism as temporary and unpleasant side effects.

Huntington's chorea is a much less common condition characterized by rapid, jerky, nonrhythmic, involuntary movements of the extremities, trunk, and/or face and by dementia. It has recently been demonstrated that this is a hereditary illness involving a disorder in chromosome no. four. The disease generally manifests itself after the age of 40.

In contrast to Huntington's chorea, *athetosis* is a disease characterized by slow, bizarre, twisting movements, especially in the arms and fingers. In these two conditions the lesion is not found in a specific subcortical nucleus (i.e., it may be in the caudate or putamen or globus pallidus). Lastly, there is *hemiballism*, which is caused by a lesion in the subthalamic nucleus. In this disease there is a violent swinging motion of the arm or leg. The causes of all three diseases are still unknown. Tragically, there is as yet no cure or relief for these sufferers, and the movements cease only in sleep.

---

*Two references on this subject are:

1. Langston, J. W. *The case of the tainted heroin. The Sciences*, 25:34–40, 1985.

2. Langston, J. W., Ballard P., et al. Chronic parkinsonism in humans due to product of meperidine analog synthesis. *Science* 219:979–980, 1983.

ACCESSORY DETAIL

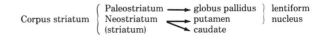

Corpus striatum { Paleostriatum ⟶ globus pallidus } lentiform nucleus
Neostriatum ⟶ putamen
(striatum) ⟵ caudate

Chapter 10

The Vestibular System

It happens to all of us—suddenly, for one reason or another, one loses one's balance, starts to fall, and immediately a reflex reaction known as the "righting mechanism" comes into play in an attempt to regain equilibrium. This sense of loss of equilibrium and the reflex mechanisms to regain and maintain it are the function of the vestibular division of the eighth cranial nerve, the acoustovestibular nerve. The vestibular system is considered part of the extrapyramidal network because it does not involve the cerebral motor cortex and its actions are reflexive.

The receptor organ is located in the inner ear and consists of two fluid-filled sacs, the *utricle* and the *sacculus*, and three fluid-filled semicircular canals (see Appendix IV, Figure 5) lying perpendicular to each other, which represent the three spatial planes (Figure 1). The fluid is *endolymph*, and suspended in it are specialized receptor cells—the *hair cells*—which are sensitive to fluid currents. When there is a shift or change of position of the head, the endolymph is set in motion. It stimulates the receptors, which transmit this information to the brain, which in turn sets off the appropriate reflex responses.

From the inner ear, primary neurons pass to the brain, with their cell bodies aggregated in the vestibular ganglion. Axons leave this ganglion and enter the brainstem, where they terminate in four vestibular nuclei situated in the area acoustica of the floor of the fourth ventricle (Figure 1). These nuclei have five major connections, which are discussed below one by one.

VESTIBULOCEREBELLAR CONNECTIONS

The cerebellum is the coordination center for motor activity and equilibrium. Therefore, from the superior and lateral vestibular nuclei, second-order (secondary) neurons pass up into the cerebellum via its inferior peduncle and terminate in the flocculonodular lobe (Figure 1). In addition, there are a few first-order axons that do not end in the vestibular nuclei but pass directly to the floccular nodulus (Figure 1). This then discharges back to the vestibular nuclei of *both sides* via the fastigial nucleus and the inferior peduncle. Thus, a cerebellar-vestibular feedback mechanism is established (Figure 1).

VESTIBULOSPINAL TRACTS

From the lateral vestibular nucleus, secondary neurons descend in the ipsilateral ventral white column and end by synapsing on lower motor neurons. These second-order neurons, which discharge reflexively to maintain equilibrium, form the lateral vestibulospinal tract (Figure 2). ("Lateral" here refers not to the fact that it originates in the lateral nucleus, but to the fact that it lies lateral to the medial vestibulospinal tract, which is discussed next.)

From the medial, superior, and inferior vestibular nuclei, second-order crossed and uncrossed neurons descend in the ventral white columns and terminate on lower motor neurons. These secondary neurons, which form the medial vestibulospinal tracts, also discharge reflexively to maintain body equilibrium (Figure 2).

VESTIBULO-OCULAR CONNECTIONS

Besides helping to maintain body equilibrium, the vestibular system also has the function of regulating eyeball movements in certain cases. For example, if one looks straight ahead and fixes one's eyes on an object and then turns one's head to the side, the appropriate eyeball muscles must contract in order for the eyes to remain "locked in" on the object. The regulation or control of this contraction is a function of the vestibular system. It works as follows: When one turns one's head, the endolymph in the semicircular canals, sacculus, and utricle is set in motion and stimulates the hair cells. This stimulus passes via the nerve and vestibular ganglion to the vestibular nuclei. We just mentioned that, from the medial, superior, and inferior nuclei, crossed and uncrossed neurons descend as the medial vestibulospinal tract. Just before descending, these neurons branch and give off axons that ascend in the pons and midbrain, where they synapse in the sixth (abducens), fourth (trochlear), and third (oculomotor) nuclei, which are all concerned with eyeball muscle movement. These ascending axons regulate the amount of eyeball muscle contraction, and form the medial longitudinal fasciculus (the MLF; Figure 2). (Some neuroanatomy books refer to the lateral vestibulospinal tract as the vestibulospinal

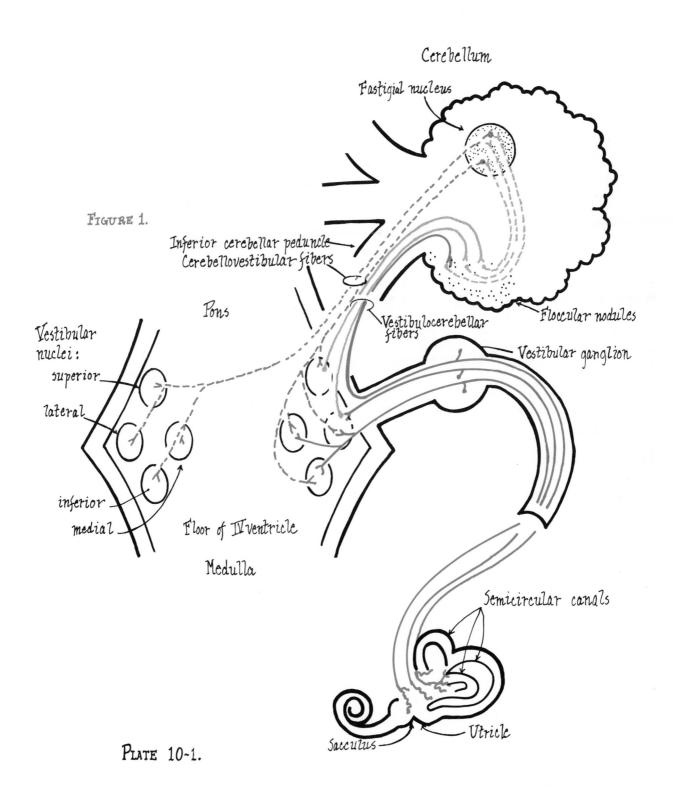

FIGURE 1.

Cerebellum

Fastigial nucleus

Inferior cerebellar peduncle
Cerebellovestibular fibers

Pons

Vestibulocerebellar fibers

Floccular nodules

Vestibular ganglion

Vestibular
nuclei:

superior

lateral

inferior

medial

Floor of IV ventricle

Medulla

Semicircular canals

Sacculus

Utricle

PLATE 10-1.

tract, whereas the medial vestibulospinal tract is called the medial longitudinal fasciculus, or MLF.)

VESTIBULOCORTICAL CONNECTIONS

We can all sense a loss of equilibrium, or dizziness, if we are spun around quickly. This sensation implies vestibular connections to the thalamus, cerebral cortex, and consciousness. However, until now no such connections have been demonstrated morphologically. Some evidence has been obtained from electrophysiologic studies, but the problem remains unsolved.

ACCESSORY PATHWAY

We mentioned above that the fastigial nucleus of the cerebellum is part of the feedback mechanism to the vestibular nuclei, which then discharge to the lower motor neurons via the lateral and medial vestibulospinal tracts. There is, in addition, another pathway to maintain equilibrium. The fastigial nucleus is connected to the descending reticular areas and nuclei of the brainstem, which then discharge to the lower motor neurons via the multisynaptic reticulospinal tract (see Figure 3 in Chapter 11, and also Chapter 18, on the reticular systems).

CLINICAL ASPECTS

Lesions of the vestibular system often produce disturbances in equilibrium and walking straight. Be-

cause this system is connected with eyeball movements, lesions in it may also produce abnormal to-and-fro movements of the eyes, known as *nystagmus*. In nystagmus the eyes are constantly moving. First they move to one side as far as they can go, and then they snap back very quickly, then again they move slowly, and so on. There is thus a slow movement to one side and a quick one to the other; the nystagmus is called left or right nystagmus according to the direction of the quick movement. Most nystagmi are horizontal in direction, but there can also be vertical nystagmus. Nystagmus is very often seen in albinos.

Normal nystagmus can be seen in persons riding on trains. While they are looking out the window, their eyes will automatically focus on an object, follow it slowly until it is out of sight, and then snap back quickly and focus on another object. This slow-fast pattern of movement is repeated. Nystagmus is a complex phenomenon, and an excellent discussion of it, as well as of the vestibular system, can be found in *A Functional Approach to Neuroanatomy*, by House and Pansky.

Another common symptom of vestibular injury is dizziness, although other conditions can also produce it. *Ménière's disease* is a disease of unknown etiology in which the patient suffers attacks of dizziness, ringing in the ears (tinnitus), and deafness.

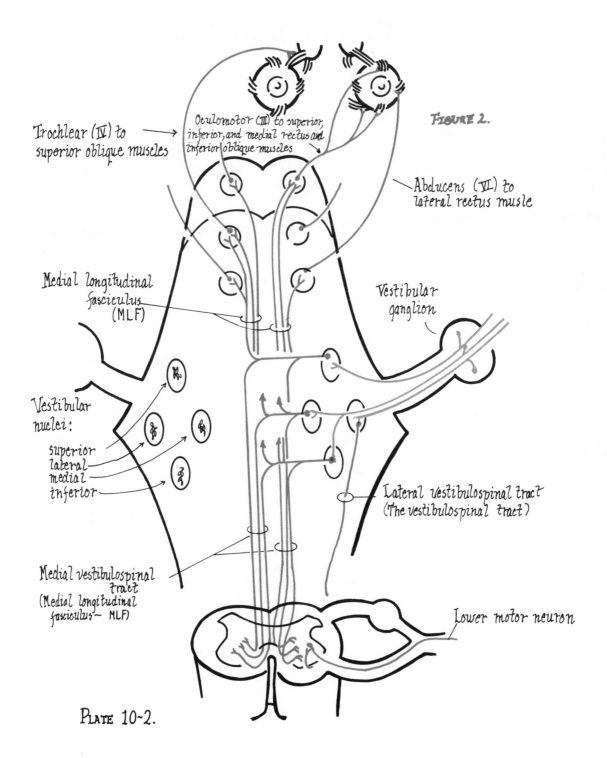

Trochlear (IV) to superior oblique muscles

Oculomotor (III) to superior, inferior, and medial rectus and inferior oblique muscles

FIGURE 2.

Abducens (VI) to lateral rectus musle

Medial longitudinal fasciculus (MLF)

Vestibular ganglion

Vestibular nuclei:

superior
lateral
medial
inferior

Lateral vestibulospinal tract (The vestibulospinal tract)

Medial vestibulospinal tract (Medial longitudinal fasciculus — MLF)

Lower motor neuron

PLATE 10-2.

Chapter 11

The Cerebellum and Its Pathways

The cerebellum (see Appendix III, Figure 4) is the control center for the coordination of voluntary muscle activity, equilibrium, and muscle tonus. It does not initiate movement; therefore, a person who has cerebellar injury does not become paralyzed. Rather, his or her movements are slow, clumsy, tremulous, and uncoordinated. The muscles may be hypertonic or hypotonic, and the person is unable to walk steadily, but tends to sway, stagger, and fall. To carry out its three important functions, the cerebellum needs to receive a steady stream of information concerning:

1. The position and state of the muscles and joints, and the amount of tonus present
2. The equilibrium state of the body
3. What "orders" are being sent to the muscles from the cerebral motor cortex.

Receiving these three information "inputs," the cerebellum is then able to integrate them and, by means of "feedback" pathways, to regulate and control motor activity, equilibrium, and muscle tonus automatically and at an unconscious level. The discussion in this chapter considers each of the information inputs separately and then presents the feedback pathways.

THE SPINOCEREBELLAR PATHWAYS

Information concerning the condition of the muscles, the amount of tonus, and the position of the body is supplied by unconscious proprioceptive fibers, whose receptors are found in joints, tendons, and muscles. The cell bodies of these neurons are situated in the dorsal root ganglion, and the axons pass into the cord, from which they can reach the cerebellum by either one of two tracts. Most of those from the lower part of the body enter the dorsal horn, where they synapse with second-order neurons (Figure 1). Some of these secondary neurons ascend on the same side, in the ventral spinocerebellar tract of the lateral columns, and enter the cerebellum through its superior peduncle. The remaining secondary axons cross over to the contralateral side, enter the ventral spinocerebellar tract there, and ascend to the cerebellum. However, before passing into the superior cerebellar peduncle they cross back to the side from which they started (Figure 1).

Proprioceptive fibers from the upper part of the body mainly use the dorsal spinocerebellar tract. Here primary neurons synapse with secondary ones in Clarke's nucleus (Figure 1), which is found only in the upper part of the spinal cord (C_8–L_2). Secondary axons pass into the lateral columns on the same side to form the dorsal spinocerebellar tract, which enters the cerebellum through the inferior cerebellar peduncle. The important thing to remember is that all spinocerebellar fibers enter the cerebellum on the same side that they entered the cord.

The dorsal and ventral spinocerebellar tracts are the main bundles supplying proprioceptive impulses to the cerebellum. There are, however, a number of others, such as the trigeminocerebellar tract from the muscles of mastication and the mandibular joint, the olivocerebellar tract, and the reticulocerebellar and arcuocerebellar tracts.

VESTIBULOCEREBELLAR TRACT

From the superior and lateral vestibular nuclei arise the fibers that supply information concerning the equilibrium state of the body. They enter through the ipsilateral (homolateral) inferior peduncle and pass to the cerebellar cortex, especially that of the flocculus (Figure 2). Phylogenetically, the flocculus is the oldest part of the cerebellum and a center for equilibrium.

CORTICOPONTOCEREBELLAR TRACTS

When the cerebral motor cortex discharges to the lower motor neurons, the cerebellum must receive information about the nature of the discharge—to what muscles it is going, how strong it is, and so on—and it gets this information through the corticopontocerebellar tracts. The fibers originate in the cerebral cortex, descend through the internal capsule, and, at the level of the pons, synapse with second-order neurons in the pontine nuclei (Figure 2). The secondary axons now cross over to the other side and enter the cerebellum through its middle peduncle.

FIGURE 1.

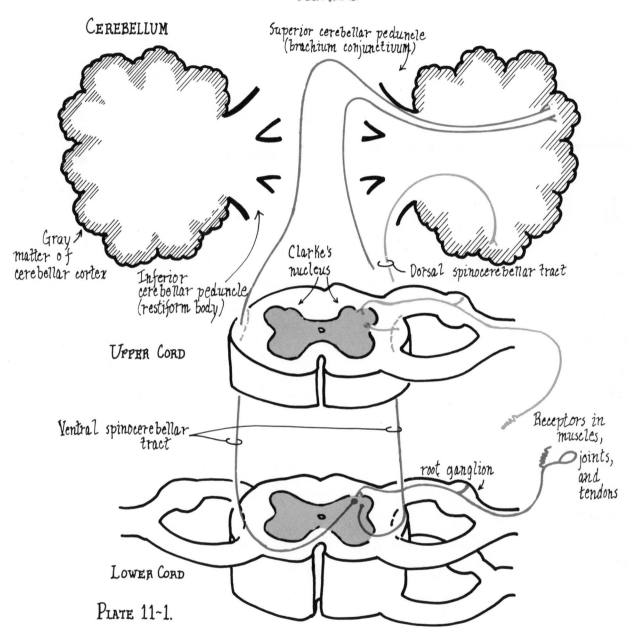

CEREBELLUM

Superior cerebellar peduncle
(brachium conjunctivum)

Gray
matter of
cerebellar cortex

Inferior
cerebellar peduncle
(restiform body)

Clarke's
nucleus

Dorsal spinocerebellar tract

UPPER CORD

Ventral spinocerebellar
tract

root ganglion

Receptors in
muscles,
joints,
and
tendons

LOWER CORD

PLATE 11~1.

FEEDBACK PATHWAYS

The cerebellum, having received information concerning muscle states, tonus, and equilibrium, as well as the nature of the motor discharge to the muscles, integrates all this input (how, we don't know) and exerts its control via the following pathways.

From the cerebellar cortex, short neurons pass to several cerebellar nuclei—the emboliform, fastigial, globose, and dentate nuclei. The last-named nucleus is the most important; it sends out fibers through the superior peduncle that decussate and then enter the red nucleus of the midbrain (Figure 3). Not surprisingly, they are called the *dentorubro fibers*, or the dentatorubrothalamic tract, because some of them bypass the red nucleus and go up to the thalamus. The red nucleus can discharge up to the thalamus, which relays the information to the cerebral motor cortex; thus the feedback circuit is completed (Figure 3). The red nucleus can also discharge down to the lower motor neuron by means of the rubrospinal tract (Figure 3) and thus can influence the corticospinal impulses at the spinal level.

The cerebellum also discharges back, directly or through the fastigial nucleus, to the vestibular nuclei. These in turn relay the stimuli to the lower motor neurons by means of the vestibulospinal tract (Figure 3).

Finally, the cerebellum can influence the lower motor neurons by discharging to the reticular area and nuclei of the pons, midbrain, and medulla, which relay the discharge by the lateral and medial reticulospinal tract (Figure 3).

CLINICAL ASPECTS

Lesions of the cerebellum or its afferent and efferent tracts produce several characteristic signs, usually on the same side of the body as the injury:

1. *Asynergia* is the loss of coordination in performing motor acts. One sees decomposition of movement; that is, it is done in jerky stages instead of smoothly.
2. *Dysmetria* is the inability to judge distance and to stop movement at a chosen spot. Thus, in reaching for an object, a patient's hand will over- or underreach it. When asked to touch the tip of the nose, the patient's finger will hit the cheek—a pass-pointing phenomenon.
3. *Adiadochokinesia* is the inability to perform rapidly alternating movements, such as pronation and supination of the hands.
4. *Intention tremor* occurs during a movement and not at rest. In Parkinson's disease one sees just the opposite—a resting tremor.
5. *Abnormal gait (ataxia)*—The patient staggers and reels. To compensate, the patient walks with the feet spread apart.
6. *Falling*—The patient has a tendency to fall, especially to the injured side.
7. *Hypotonia*—The muscles are floppy and weak, but may be hypertonic in some cases.
8. *Dysphonia* is a slurred, explosive speech.
9. *Nystagmus* may be present.

Not all these signs or symptoms are present in every case of cerebellar damage. To test, ask the patient to perform the various movements described above, and check for their presence or absence.

Medulloblastoma (Appendix III, Figure 16) is the most common CNS tumor in children and is found mostly in the 4–8 age group. It is situated in the vermis or roof of the fourth ventricle, and the first characteristic signs are ataxia (i.e., stumbling gait) and/or frequent unexplained falls. This tumor is very radiosensitive, and with correct therapy there is a 5-year survival time in more than 60% of cases. Medulloblastoma is never found in adults.

FIGURE 2.

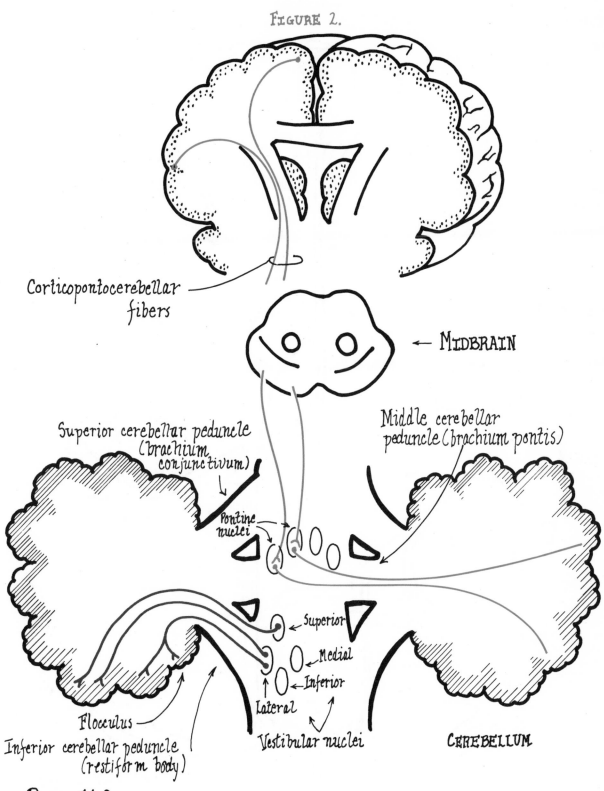

Corticopontocerebellar
fibers

← MIDBRAIN

Superior cerebellar peduncle
(brachium
conjunctivum)

Middle cerebellar
peduncle (brachium pontis)

Pontine
nuclei

Superior

Medial

Inferior

Lateral

Vestibular nuclei

CEREBELLUM

Flocculus

Inferior cerebellar peduncle
(restiform body)

PLATE 11-2.

FIGURE 3.

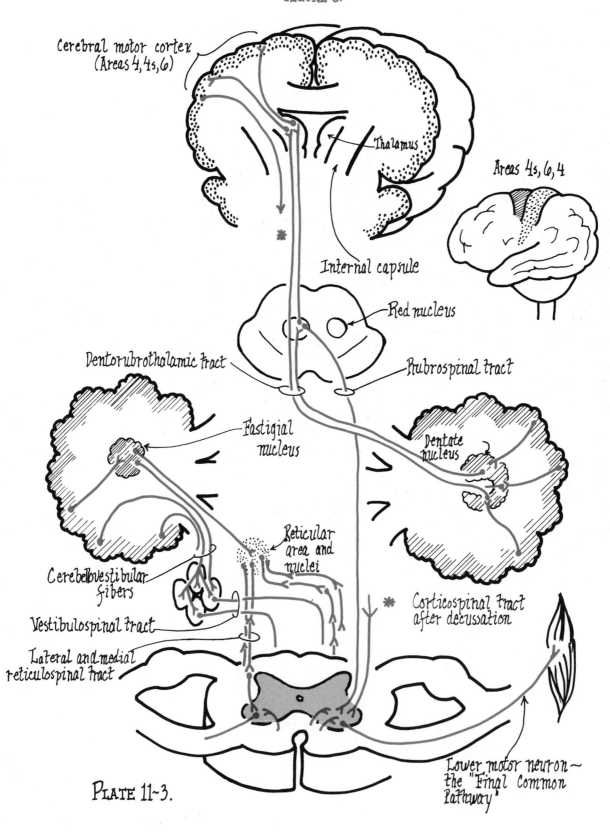

Cerebral motor cortex
(Areas 4, 4s, 6)

Thalamus

Areas 4s, 6, 4

Internal capsule

Red nucleus

Dentorubrothalamic tract

Rubrospinal tract

Fastigial nucleus

Dentate nucleus

Cerebellovestibular fibers

Reticular area and nuclei

Vestibulospinal tract

Corticospinal tract after decussation

Lateral and medial reticulospinal tract

Lower motor neuron — the "Final Common Pathway"

PLATE 11~3.

Chapter 12

The Autonomic Nervous System

The autonomic nervous system (ANS), which is also known as the visceral or vegetative nervous system, stimulates and controls structures not under conscious control. If, for example, you are suddenly told that you're getting a surprise exam, your heart rate will probably increase, your mouth will go dry, you'll get "butterflies" in your stomach, and you'll start sweating—all automatic reactions to a stress situation. The autonomic nervous system stimulates three types of tissues: cardiac muscle, most glands, and all smooth muscle (that found in many organs and structures). The autonomic system is divided into two parts: the *sympathetic* nervous system and the *parasympathetic* nervous system, both of which supply (with two or three exceptions) the same organs and structures. However, the two systems are antagonistic to each other. For example, sympathetic stimulation of the heart results in an increased pulse rate, whereas parasympathetic stimulation slows it down. Sympathetic discharge results in dilation of the pupils, whereas parasympathetic stimulation produces constriction. The two systems are constantly discharging to the structures they supply, but there is a balance between them (Figure 1a). *This balance can be changed in either of two ways: by increasing the amount of stimulus in one part of the system* (Figure 1b) *or by decreasing the amount of discharge in the other* (Figure 1c). This very important principle forms the basis of much of neuropharmacology and is discussed later in greater detail. It can be remembered easily as the "water tap" principle. If you have the hot (sympathetic) and cold (parasympathetic) taps open equally, then lukewarm water flows. Now if you want the water warmer you can either *open the hot water tap more or close the cold one*, and vice versa if you want the water colder.

THE SYMPATHETIC NERVOUS SYSTEM

The sympathetic nervous system is the one that dominates when a person is in a stress situation, be it physical or psychological. In both instances one feels threatened, and the body automatically reacts by preparing for "fight or flight." In these conditions the muscles will work harder, will need more oxygen, and will use more energy. Therefore, one breathes faster and the bronchioles open up for quicker and greater passage of air; the heart beats stronger and faster to increase cardiac output; the arteries to the heart and voluntary muscles dilate, thereby bringing more blood to them; the arteries to the skin and peripheral areas of the body constrict, thereby shunting more blood to the active muscles (as a result the skin feels cold); the liver secretes glycogen for quick supply of energy; peristalsis slows down, because the body has no energy or time for digestion; the pupils dilate to get a better view of the surroundings; the hair "stands on end"; and one sweats. The last two responses are interesting evolutionary carryovers of more primitive defense reactions. The hairs of a cat that is threatened by a dog stand up, so that if the dog attempts to bite the body it gets a mouthful of hairs instead. As for sweating, did you ever try to grab and hold a person who is wet and slippery?

The sympathetic nervous system is based on a two-neuron pathway. The cell bodies of the first neurons are located in the lateral gray horn of the spinal cord, which is situated only between the first thoracic and the third lumbar (T_1–L_3) segments (Figure 2; the system is also called the thoracolumbar outflow). The axons leave the cord via the ventral roots and enter the sympathetic trunk. The sympathetic trunk is made up of a series of ganglia and axon fibers on each side of the vertebral column that extends from the neck to the sacrum. It is also referred to as the paravertebral chain ganglia or the sympathetic chain. The question is: How do the primary axons that exit at T_1 reach the glands and smooth-muscled structures up in the head? After entering the sympathetic trunk, the axons ascend until they reach the superior cervical ganglion in the upper region of the neck (Figure 2). Here they synapse with secondary neurons, which go out and innervate the glands and other structures. The first neuron is called the *preganglionic neuron*, and its axon is myelinated; the second is the *postganglionic neuron*, and its axon is unmyelinated. This postganglionic axon reaches its destination by leaving the superior cervical ganglion and wrapping itself around the arteries that supply the innervated structures. It thus "hitches a ride" on the arteries until it comes to the glands and smooth-muscled structures, where it then peels off to innervate them (Figure 2).

Cell bodies of sympathetics destined to supply

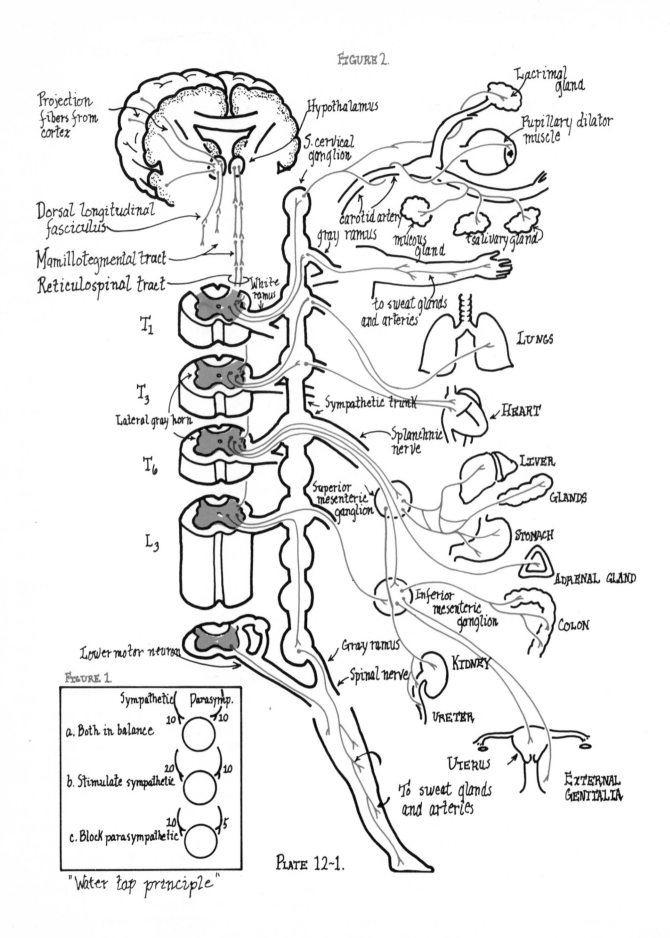

FIGURE 2.

Projection fibers from cortex

Hypothalamus

S. cervical ganglion

Lacrimal gland

Pupillary dilator muscle

carotid artery

gray ramus

mucous gland

salivary gland

Dorsal longitudinal fasciculus

Mamillotegmental tract

Reticulospinal tract

White ramus

to sweat glands and arteries

T_1

T_3

Lateral gray horn

T_6

Sympathetic trunk

Splanchnic nerve

Superior mesenteric ganglion

LUNGS

HEART

LIVER

GLANDS

L_3

STOMACH

ADRENAL GLAND

Inferior mesenteric ganglion

COLON

Lower motor neuron

FIGURE 1.

Gray ramus

Spinal nerve

KIDNEY

URETER

UTERUS

EXTERNAL GENITALIA

To sweat glands and arteries

	Sympathetic	Parasymp.
a. Both in balance	10	10
b. Stimulate sympathetic	20	10
c. Block parasympathetic	10	5

PLATE 12~1.

"Water tap principle"

40

the heart and lungs are situated in the lateral gray horn of segments T_1–T_5. The axons leave the cord and enter the chain ganglia, where they synapse with postganglionic neurons. The axons of the latter leave the chain ganglia and form specific nerves that reach the heart and lungs (Figure 2).

Those sympathetics that supply the abdominal viscera are found in the lateral horn of T_5–T_{12}. Their axons enter the chain ganglia, but do not synapse there. Rather, they pass through it and leave to form distinct nerves, the greater and lesser splanchnics, which terminate in the superior and inferior mesenteric ganglions of the abdomen. The postganglionic axons leave and form a net-like plexus that spreads out over the arteries to reach the various organs. Some of the preganglionic axons pass to the adrenal gland, the medullary cells of which are the postganglionic neurons that are specialized to secrete the hormone adrenaline (Figure 2).

Most of the preganglionic nerve cell bodies to the pelvic organs are located in the lateral horn of spinal segments L_1–L_3 (Figure 2). Their axons enter the sympathetic chain, pass through it without synapsing, and descend to end in the inferior mesenteric ganglion. From here the postganglionics fan out to supply the urinary and genital organs, as well as the descending and sigmoid colon and the rectum.

Accessory Details

The preganglionic sympathetic axons are myelinated and are therefore white. They leave the cord and peel off from the spinal nerve to form the white *rami communicantes*, which links up the spinal nerves with the sympathetic ganglia (Figure 2). The postganglionic axons are unmyelinated and therefore appear gray. Many rejoin the spinal nerves through the gray rami communicantes and pass out to supply the sweat glands and peripheral arteries of the head, upper extremity, the trunk, and the lower limbs (Figure 2).

The chemical transmitter between the postganglionic sympathetic axons and the structures they innervate is not acetylcholine, but adrenaline. If a patient is given a shot of adrenaline, the reaction is the same as if the sympathetic nervous system had discharged. Consequently, this system is also called the *adrenergic nervous system.* There are drugs that block the parasympathetic system, resulting in an imbalance between the two parts of the autonomic nervous system, and what one sees is similar in many ways to what happens when the sympathetics discharge (Figure 1c).

THE PARASYMPATHETIC NERVOUS SYSTEM

This system is also based on a two-neuron pathway, consisting of preganglionic and postganglionic neurons. However, there are great physiologic, anatomic, and pharmacologic differences between the two systems. Whereas the sympathetic nervous system is dominant in stress situations, the parasympathetic is most active when a person is relaxed and resting; the heart beat slows down, peristalsis and other digestive functions are active, and so on.

The chemical transmitter between the postganglionic parasympathetic axons and the structures they innervate is acetylcholine. Thus, if one gives a patient such a drug, the reaction resembles parasympathetic discharge.

As for the anatomy, the preganglionic cell bodies are located in the brainstem and in the gray matter of the cord in the sacral region. Thus another name for this system is the cranial-sacral outflow. In the brainstem the cell bodies are aggregated in several specific nuclei, and the axons join cranial nerves III, VII, IX, and X. Being components of these nerves, they exit with them, pass out to the different regions, and, very near their destinations, enter specific named ganglia. Here the preganglionic axons synapse with short postganglionic fibers that innervate glands, the heart, and structures having smooth muscle. In many cases the ganglia are situated near, on, or within the structures innervated, and the postganglionic fibers are microscopic.

At the level of the superior colliculus of the midbrain, preganglionic cell bodies are located in the *Edinger-Westphal nucleus* (Figure 3). The axons join the lower motor fibers of the oculomotor nerve (cranial nerve III), and together they leave the midbrain and course out to the eyeball (Figure 3). Near it, the preganglionic axons peel off and enter the ciliary ganglion, where they synapse with postganglionic neurons. These send out short axons to the pupillary constrictor muscle.

The preganglionic cell bodies associated with the facial nerve (cranial nerve VII) are situated in the superior salivary nucleus, and their axons pass out to the sphenopalatine (pterygopalatine) and submandibular (submaxillary) ganglia (Figure 3). From here the postganglionic axons course out to the lacrimal gland, as well as to the sublingual and submandibular glands.

As for cranial nerve IX, the glossopharyngeal, its preganglionic cell bodies are in the inferior salivatory nucleus, and the axons go out to the otic gan-

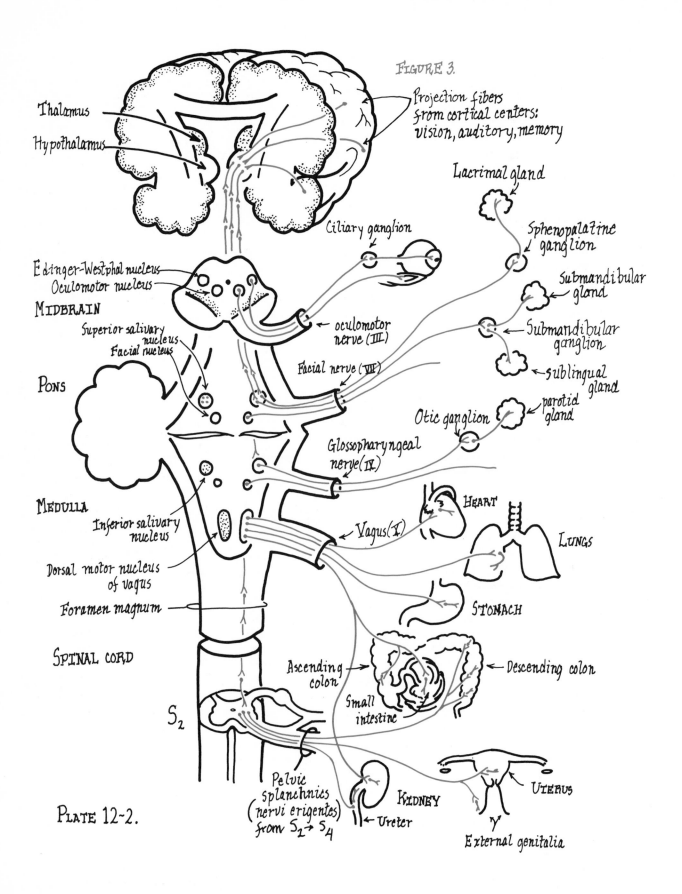

FIGURE 3.

Thalamus

Hypothalamus

Projection fibers
from cortical centers:
vision, auditory, memory

Lacrimal gland

Ciliary ganglion

Sphenopalatine
ganglion

Edinger-Westphal nucleus
Oculomotor nucleus

MIDBRAIN

Submandibular
gland

oculomotor
nerve (III)

Submandibular
ganglion

Superior salivary
nucleus
Facial nucleus

PONS

Facial nerve (VII)

sublingual
gland

Otic ganglion

parotid
gland

Glossopharyngeal
nerve (IX)

HEART

LUNGS

MEDULLA

Vagus (X)

Inferior salivary
nucleus

Dorsal motor nucleus
of vagus

STOMACH

Foramen magnum

SPINAL CORD

Ascending
colon

Descending colon

Small
intestine

S_2

Pelvic
splanchnics
(nervi erigentes)
from $S_2 \rightarrow S_4$

KIDNEY

Ureter

UTERUS

External genitalia

PLATE 12-2.

glion, which sends out postganglionic fibers to the parotid gland (Figure 3).

The vagus nerve (cranial nerve X) is the most important cranial nerve because most of its fibers are parasympathetic neurons that innervate the heart, lungs, and all the abdominal viscera up to the left colic flexure. The preganglionic cell bodies are aggregated in the dorsal motor nucleus of the vagus, and the axons pass out and terminate in ganglia situated near or in the walls of the above-mentioned organs (Figure 3). From these ganglia, postganglionic neurons innervate the structures.

The descending colon and the genital and urinary systems are supplied by the sacral outflow. Here the preganglionic cell bodies are situated in the lateral area of the gray matter of spinal segments S_2–S_4. The axons leave through the ventral roots and soon separate from the spinal nerve to form the pelvic splanchnic nerves or nervi erigentes, which reach the mural ganglia of the descending colon, ureter, and genital organs (Figure 3).

Accessory Detail

The hypothalamus is the control and integrative center for the autonomic nervous system, and its actions are automatic and not regularly subject to conscious control. (The hypothalamus is part of the diencephalon and lies below the thalamus on either side of the third ventricle (Figure 3).) It receives fiber bundles mainly from higher cortical centers, such as vision, auditory, personality, etc., and then discharges the appropriate impulses down the cord to the sympathetic or parasympathetic preganglionic neurons. It does this by means of the dorsal longitudinal fasciculus, the mamillotegmental tract, and the multisynaptic reticulospinal tract (see Chapters 17 and 18 on the reticular formation and the hypothalamus).

Pain pathways from the viscera are poorly understood, but it is generally accepted that the impulses travel via the autonomic nerves. Thus the system is afferent as well as efferent.

CLINICAL ASPECTS

The action of adrenergic drugs (e.g., adrenaline (epinephrine) and noradrenaline (norepinephrine)) mimics sympathetic activity. They are also known as sympathomimetics and are used primarily in hospitals to deal with cases of falling blood pressure and cardiac arrest. They are also used to dilate the bronchioles in asthma and in cases of anaphylactic shock. Adrenergic drugs are also injected at sites of local anesthesia to constrict blood vessels, thereby slowing the rate of anesthetic absorption and increasing the duration of its effect. Sympathetic antagonists are those drugs that block sympathetic activity. In recent years they have become among the most important and widely used drugs, primarily in the treatment of hypertension.

The action of cholinergic (or parasympathomimetic) drugs duplicates parasympathetic activity. These have relatively little use in medical practice, being employed in cases where smooth muscle activation is needed (e.g., to stimulate an incontinent bladder).

The parasympathetic blocking agents have a wider use and among the most common is atropine (belladonna*), which causes marked pupillary dilation and is therefore used by ophthalmologists when they want to take a good look at the eye. However before administering atropine one must make sure that the patient doesn't have glaucoma because dilating the pupil in such a patient can precipitate occulogyric attack with a great increase in ocular pressure and subsequent damage to the retina.

---

*This drug got its name from the fact that, during the Renaissance, women used it to dilate their pupils in an attempt to make their eyes more beautiful (*bella donna* is Italian for "beautiful lady"), even though it seriously blurred their vision.

Chapter 13

Cranial Nerves

The 12 pairs of cranial nerves, which we have already discussed in passing in previous chapters, are considered in detail here. These nerves can be grouped in several ways, the first according to their central location (see figures in this chapter and also Appendix II). Cranial nerves I and II, the olfactory and optic nerves, are connected to the telencephalon and diencephalon, respectively. Nerves III and IV, the oculomotor and trochlear nerves, are connected with the midbrain; the trigeminal (V), the abducens (VI), and the facial (VII) nerves are located in the pons; the remaining nerves (VIII, IX, X, XI, and XII) are associated with the medulla. It is important to know this location plan because if a patient exhibits signs of a specific cranial nerve injury, then the site of the lesion can be pinpointed.

Another way to group cranial nerves is according to their functional neuronal components. Some have only sensory neurons; and they are (Figure 1a):

I, the *olfactory* nerve, concerned with smell (see Chapter 16)

II, the *optic* nerve, which deals with vision (see Chapter 15)

VIII, the *acoustovestibular* nerve, concerned with hearing and equilibrium (see Chapters 10 and 14).

Other cranial nerves are composed only of motor neurons to voluntary muscles; they are (Figure 1b):

IV, the *trochlear* nerve, which innervates the superior oblique muscle of the eyeball. If the nerve or its nucleus is damaged, the muscle will be paralyzed and there will be difficulty in turning the affected eye downward and laterally.

VI, the *abducens* nerve, which innervates the lateral rectus muscle of the eyeball. If this nerve or its nucleus is injured, the muscle becomes paralyzed, and the patient can't turn the eye laterally. In time, the unopposed medial rectus causes the eye to be pulled medially, thus producing a medial strabismus (squint).

XI, the *accessory* nerve, which innervates two important muscles outside the head: the trapezius and the sternocleidomastoid muscles. These two neck muscles are also supplied by spinal nerves; thus, if the accessory nerve or its nucleus is damaged, the muscle will still function partially. However, the patient will have difficulty shrugging the shoulder on the affected side and turning the head to the opposite side.

XII, the *hypoglossal* nerve, which supplies all the muscles of the tongue. Again, if this nerve or its nucleus is damaged, then the muscles on the affected side become paralyzed, and the tongue, when protruded, will deviate to the paralyzed side. The reason for this is that tongue muscles are so arranged that, if one side is paralyzed, then, upon protrusion, the muscles on the unparalyzed side pull the tongue over to the paralyzed side.

The remaining cranial nerves (III, V, VII, IX, and X) have mixed functional neuronal components (Figure 1c). Each of these mixed cranial nerves is discussed below in detail.

THE OCULOMOTOR NERVE (III)

The motor nucleus of the oculomotor nerve is located in the midbrain below the aqueduct of Sylvius at the level of the superior colliculus (Figure 2 and Appendix II, Plate X). From it emerge voluntary motor fibers (lower motor neurons), which leave the brainstem at the interpeduncular fossa and pass into the orbit through the superior orbital fissure. Here they supply the following four eyeball muscles: the superior rectus, inferior rectus, and medial rectus muscles, and the inferior oblique muscle. In addition, they innervate the levator palpebrae superioris, which is responsible for lifting the upper eyelid.

The Edinger-Westphal nucleus is the parasympathetic nucleus of the oculomotor nerve and is situated just dorsal to the motor nucleus (Figure 2). Preganglionic fibers leave it, join the voluntary motor fibers, and pass out to the orbit. There the parasympathetic fibers separate, and most of them terminate in the ciliary ganglion (Figure 2). Here they synapse with postganglionic fibers that stimulate the sphincter pupillae muscle, causing the pupil to constrict. Other postganglionic fibers from the ciliary ganglion pass to the ciliary muscle, which is concerned with lens accommodation for near vision.

Clinical Aspects

Because the oculomotor nucleus receives a bilateral upper motor neuron supply via the corticobulbar tract (Chapter 8), one rarely sees an upper motor (a supranuclear) lesion that affects this nerve. However, if the oculomotor nerve is damaged, there is a lower motor neuron paralysis of the muscles it supplies, and the eyeball is pulled laterally and down-

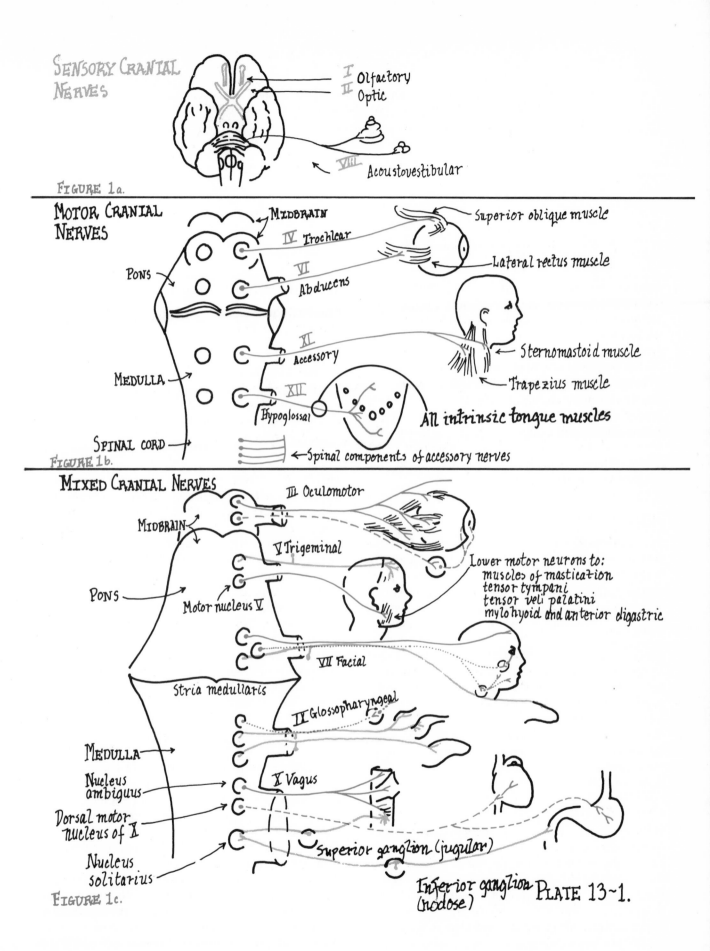

SENSORY CRANIAL NERVES

I Olfactory
II Optic

VIII Acoustovestibular

FIGURE 1a.

MOTOR CRANIAL NERVES

MIDBRAIN

IV Trochlear

Superior oblique muscle

PONS

VI Abducens

Lateral rectus muscle

XI Accessory

Sternomastoid muscle

Trapezius muscle

MEDULLA

XII Hypoglossal

All intrinsic tongue muscles

SPINAL CORD

Spinal components of accessory nerves

FIGURE 1b.

MIXED CRANIAL NERVES

III Oculomotor

MIDBRAIN

V Trigeminal

PONS

Motor nucleus V

Lower motor neurons to:
muscles of mastication
tensor tympani
tensor veli palatini
mylohyoid and anterior digastric

VII Facial

Stria medullaris

IX Glossopharyngeal

MEDULLA

X Vagus

Nucleus ambiguus

Dorsal motor nucleus of X

Nucleus solitarius

superior ganglion (jugular)

Inferior ganglion (nodose)

PLATE 13~1.

FIGURE 1c.

45

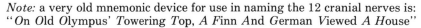
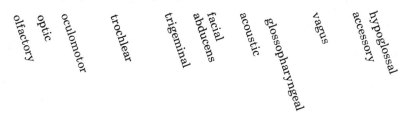
ward by the unopposed lateral rectus muscle (supplied by the abducens nerve) and the superior oblique muscle (supplied by the trochlear). Because the levator palpebrae is paralyzed, the upper eyelid droops—a condition known as *ptosis*. In addition, the parasympathetic fibers will be damaged and, as a result, the sphincter pupillae will be paralyzed. The dilator pupillae, supplied by the sympathetics, is now unopposed, and consequently the pupil is widely dilated and cannot constrict (in other words, there is a "fixed pupil"). Also, oculomotor nerve damage causes difficulty in visual accommodation because the ciliary muscle is paralyzed.

THE TRIGEMINAL NERVE (V)

This trigeminal nerve has general sensory fibers as well as voluntary motor neurons. The sensory fibers (Chapter 6) convey general sensations of pain, temperature, touch, pressure, and proprioception from the face, cornea, mouth, nose sinuses, tongue, teeth, meninges, outer surface of the eardrum, and temporomandibular joint. The motor component consists of voluntary or lower motor neurons that supply the four muscles of mastication—the temporalis, the masseter, the lateral, and the medial pterygoids (Figure 1c). In addition, the trigeminal motor fibers innervate the anterior belly of the digastric, the mylohyoid, and the tensor tympani and tensor veli palatini muscles. The motor nucleus of the trigeminal nerve is located in the pons near the main sensory nucleus.

Clinical Aspects

If the entire nerve is cut or damaged, there will be a complete loss of sensation in the facial area on the same side, as well as a lower motor neuron lesion that produces difficulty in chewing and speaking. Because this nerve receives a bilateral innervation from the cerebral cortex, one rarely sees cases of upper motor neuron lesions (see also "Clinical Aspects" in Chapter 6).

THE FACIAL NERVE (VII)

The facial nerve is a more complex nerve that has three major components:

1. Special sensory fibers for taste from the anterior two-thirds of the tongue
2. Parasympathetic fibers to the sublingual, submandibular (submaxillary), and lacrimal glands
3. Voluntary motor fibers to all the muscles of facial expression.

The taste receptors are located on the anterior two-thirds of the tongue, and their fibers pass back to the brainstem (Figure 4). In their course, they merge with the lingual branch of the trigeminal nerve, but then they separate from it to form the nerve known as the *chorda tympani*. This nerve enters the skull through a small fissure and passes into the temporal bone, in which is situated the geniculate ganglion. Here are located the cell bodies of the taste neurons, the axons of which pass into the pons and end in the nucleus solitarius (Figures 4 and 4a). From this nucleus second-order ascending gustatory tracts arise that reach conscious levels; however, their exact course is unknown. In addition, there are reflex pathways for taste sensations. For example, when one tastes something pleasant there is a reflex salivation, and this pathway involves the parasympathetic component of both the seventh and ninth cranial nerves. From the nucleus solitarius internuncials pass down to the superior salivary nucleus and synapse with preganglionic neurons (Figure 4). Their axons leave the pons, enter the internal auditory meatus, and travel through the geniculate ganglion. They then separate from the rest of the facial nerves fibers to form the chorda tympani, which merges with the lingual nerve. After "hitching a ride" with the lingual nerve, the preganglionic parasympathetics again separate and terminate in the submandibular (submaxillary) ganglion. Here they synapse with the postganglionic neurons, which stimulate the

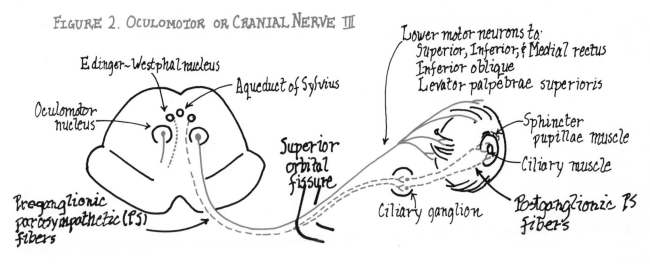

FIGURE 2. OCULOMOTOR OR CRANIAL NERVE III

Edinger-Westphal nucleus

Oculomotor nucleus

Aqueduct of Sylvius

Lower motor neurons to:
Superior, Inferior, & Medial rectus
Inferior oblique
Levator palpebrae superioris

Superior orbital fissure

Sphincter pupillae muscle

Ciliary muscle

Preganglionic parasympathetic (PS) fibers

Ciliary ganglion

Postganglionic PS fibers

FIGURE 3. GLOSSOPHARYNGEAL OR CRANIAL NERVE IX

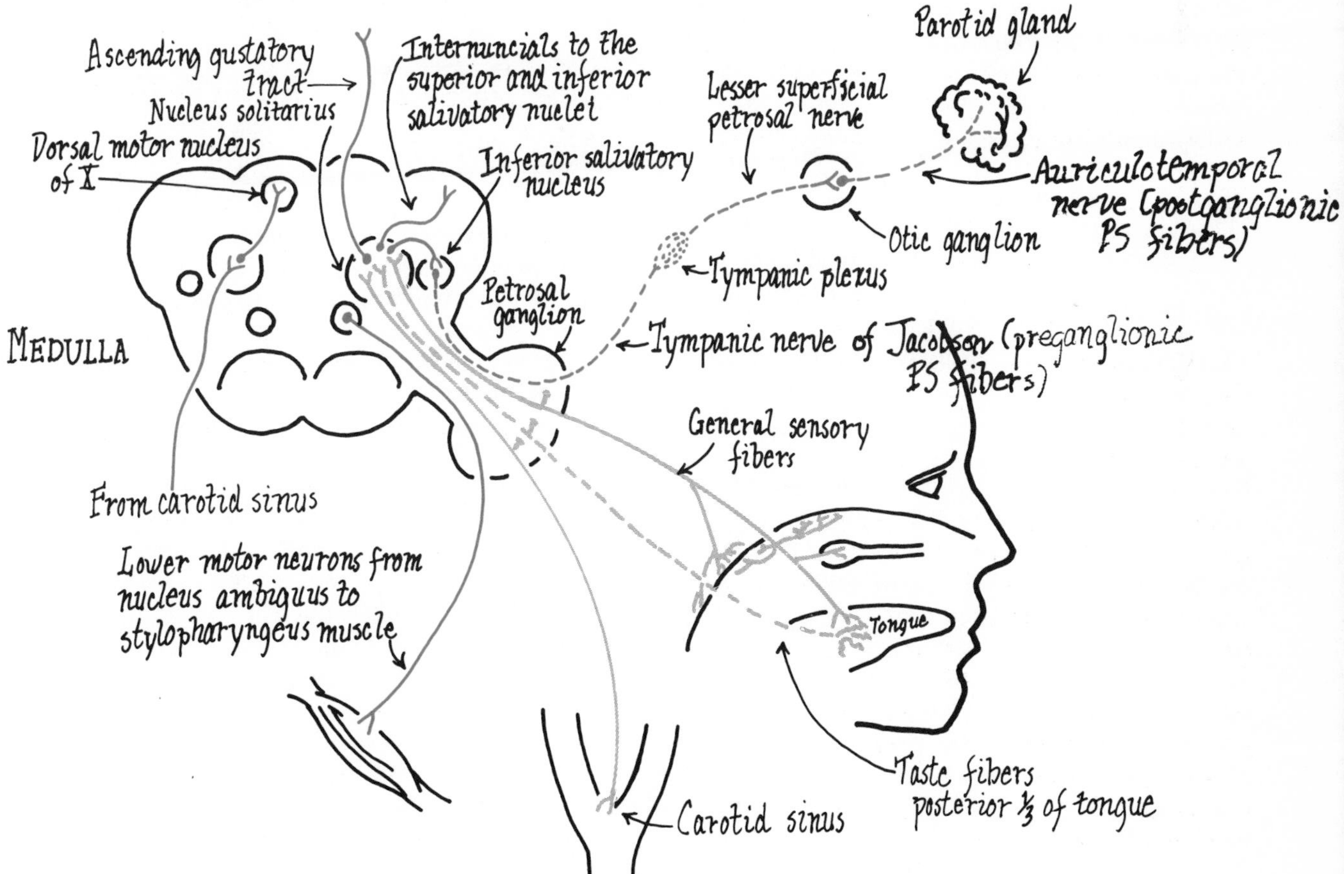

Ascending gustatory tract

Nucleus solitarius

Dorsal motor nucleus of IX

Internuncials to the superior and inferior salivatory nuclei

Inferior salivatory nucleus

Parotid gland

Lesser superficial petrosal nerve

Auriculotemporal nerve (postganglionic PS fibers)

Otic ganglion

Tympanic plexus

MEDULLA

Petrosal ganglion

Tympanic nerve of Jacobson (preganglionic PS fibers)

General sensory fibers

From carotid sinus

Lower motor neurons from nucleus ambiguus to stylopharyngeus muscle

Tongue

Carotid sinus

Taste fibers posterior ⅓ of tongue

PLATE 13-2.

47

submandibular and sublingual salivary glands. From the superior salivatory nucleus other preganglionic parasympathetic neurons follow a different course and reach the sphenopalatine (pterygopalatine) ganglion, where they synapse with postganglionic neurons (Figure 4). These postganglionic neurons follow a complicated pathway to reach the lacrimal gland and the mucus-secreting cells of the nose and mouth (Figure 4).

The last major component of the facial nerve is voluntary motor fibers to all the muscles of facial expression. Their nucleus is found in the tegmentum of the pons below the nucleus of cranial nerve VI (Figure 4). The emerging motor fibers pass up and loop around the abducens nucleus, causing a bulge on the floor of the fourth ventricle that is known as the *facial colliculus*. These motor fibers then join the rest of the components and enter the internal auditory meatus. After the taste and parasympathetic neurons have separated from the main bundle, the remaining voluntary motor fibers leave the skull at the stylomastoid foramen and separate into five main branches that supply all the muscles of facial expression, as well as the posterior belly of the digastric muscle. Within the temporal bone some motor fibers supply the stapedius muscle of the middle ear, which acts as a "brake" on the hearing apparatus and prevents hyperacusis (i.e., normal sounds heard abnormally loud on the affected side).

Clinical Aspects

The most common pathologic condition involving the seventh cranial nerve is Bell's palsy. In this condition, nerve damage of unknown etiology quickly results in a characteristic lower motor neuron paralysis and of varying degrees of severity of the muscles of facial expression on the affected side. The person is unable to close the affected eye because the orbicularis oculi muscle is paralyzed. The unopposed muscles on the unaffected side contract and pull the mouth up in a characteristic grotesque grin. The lesions may affect the stapedius muscle, and the patient will suffer from hyperacusis. In addition, there may be a partial loss of taste and salivation, and a total loss of lacrimation on the affected side.

From a treatment point of view there is no cure, but in most cases the condition disappears slowly over a period of time ranging from weeks to months. Of prime importance is the psychological support given to the patient throughout the episode.

It is believed that in some cases a herpes simplex virus causes inflamation (neuritis) of the nerve within the temporal bone, and the resulting edema presses on the nerve causing axonal damage and symptoms.

Because the lower part of the motor nucleus receives its upper motor neuron supply only from the contralateral corticobulbar tract (Chapter 8), an upper motor or supranuclear lesion will produce a contralateral spastic paralysis of the muscles of the lower half of the face. Because the muscles of the upper half of the face have a bilateral nerve supply, the patient with such a lesion can still close the eyes and wrinkle the brow. These two actions help differentiate between Bell's palsy, which is a lower motor neuron paralysis, and an upper motor neuron lesion.

THE GLOSSOPHARYNGEAL NERVE (IX)

The glossopharyngeal nerve also has three major components:

1. Special sensory taste neurons from the posterior third of the tongue
2. Parasympathetic fibers to the parotid gland
3. General sensory neurons from the auditory tube, the back of the tongue, the inner surface of the tympanic membrane, the pharynx, and the carotid sinus.

On the surface of the posterior third of the tongue are situated the taste receptors of the ninth cranial nerve. The cell bodies of these neurons are located in the petrosal ganglion (Figure 3), and their axons end in the nucleus solitarius, which extends down from the pons into the medulla. Here they synapse with cell bodies whose ascending gustatory fibers eventually reach conscious levels, but their pathway and final cortical localization are unclear. As is the case with the seventh nerve, there are also reflex arcs involving taste. From the solitarius nucleus, short internuncials pass to the inferior salivatory nucleus and synapse with preganglionic parasympathetic neurons. The axons of the latter leave the medulla along with the other glossopharyngeal fibers, but then separate and follow a long course (Figure 3) to reach the otic ganglion. Here they synapse with postganglionic parasympathetic neurons that stimulate the parotid salivary gland. Other internuncials from the nucleus solitarius pass up and synapse in the superior salivary nu-

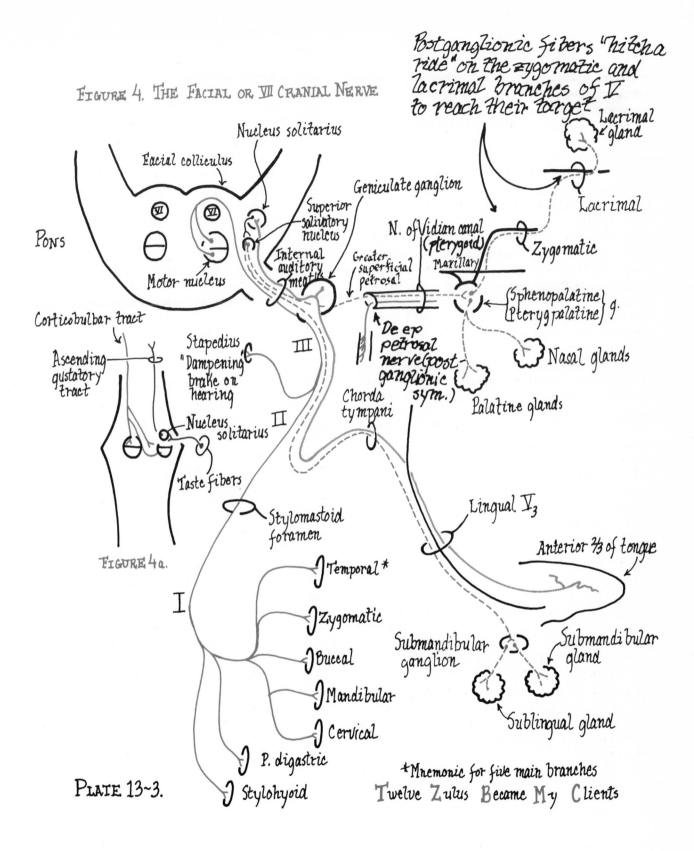

FIGURE 4. THE FACIAL OR VII CRANIAL NERVE

Postganglionic fibers "hitch a ride" on the zygomatic and lacrimal branches of V to reach their target

Lacrimal gland

Lacrimal

Nucleus solitarius

Facial colliculus

Geniculate ganglion

Superior salivatory nucleus

N. of Vidian canal (pterygoid)

Zygomatic

Maxillary

Pons

VI   VI

Internal auditory meatus

Greater superficial petrosal

{Sphenopalatine} g. {Pterygpalatine}

Motor nucleus

Deep petrosal nerve (post-ganglionic sym.)

Nasal glands

Corticobulbar tract

III

II

Palatine glands

Ascending gustatory tract

Stapedius "Dampening brake on hearing"

Chorda tympani

Lingual V₃

Anterior ⅔ of tongue

Nucleus solitarius

II

Taste fibers

FIGURE 4a.

Stylomastoid foramen

I

Temporal *

Submandibular ganglion

Submandibular gland

Zygomatic

Buccal

Mandibular

Sublingual gland

Cervical

P. digastric

*Mnemonic for five main branches

PLATE 13~3.

Stylohyoid

Twelve Zulus Became My Clients

49

cleus, the fibers of which reach the sublingual and submandibular glands (see the discussion of the facial nerve above).

The last major component of the glossopharyngeal nerve is the general sensory component, involving pain, pressure, touch, and temperature. The receptors are found in the Eustachian tube, the middle ear, the inner surface of the tympanic membrane, the uvula, the carotid sinus, and the nasal and oral pharynx. The fibers from these areas pass back to the inferior or petrosal ganglia, which house their cell bodies, and terminate in the nucleus solitarius. Here they synapse with neurons of various tracts. Some of these ascend to consciousness, and others set off important reflexes, such as the gag reflex (see "Clinical Aspects"). Another example involves the carotid sinus, which is sensitive to blood pressure changes. A rise in blood pressure stimulates this receptor, which fires off a compensatory reflex. From the nucleus solitarius an internuncial neuron passes to the dorsal motor nucleus of the vagus nerve (cranial nerve X) and synapses with a parasympathetic neuron. The latter descends to the heart and stimulates it to slow down the heart rate, thus lowering the blood pressure.

The glossopharyngeal nerve also has voluntary motor neurons that stimulate the stylopharyngeus muscle (Figure 3).

Clinical Aspects

If the uvula or oral pharynx is touched, a gag or swallowing reflex is set off, and the trachea is closed by the epiglottis. However, when a patient is under general gas anesthesia, this reflex does not work. Furthermore, the unconscious patient often vomits. It is therefore *absolutely imperative* that, before general surgery, *no food or liquid be given* to the patient for 8 to 12 hours before the procedure; otherwise the patient may vomit while unconscious, and the acid contents from the stomach will enter the now wide-open trachea and lungs—with a fatal result.

THE VAGUS NERVE (X)

The vagus nerve, a vital nerve, has three major components:

1. Parasympathetic fibers to all the autonomic structures of the chest and abdomen up to the left colic flexure (e.g., heart, coronary arteries, bronchioles, stomach, small and large intestine arterioles, glands). (Chapter 12, Figure 3)
2. Voluntary motor fibers to the muscles of larynx and pharynx involved in talking and swallowing.
3. General sensory fibers from all the larynx, the viscera, the carotid body (a chemoreceptor), the carotid sinus, the dura of the posterior cranial fossa, and the lower part of the pharynx. The cell bodies are located in the nodose or inferior ganglia, and the axons end in the nucleus solitarius (Figure 1c).

The parasympathetic fibers arise from the dorsal motor nucleus of the vagus nerve, which is found in the floor of the fourth ventricle of the medulla, just lateral to the hypoglossal nucleus (Appendix II, Plate XIV). The preganglionic fibers leave and descend into the chest and abdomen, where they synapse in ganglia that are situated on or in the organs that are innervated (Figure 1c of this chapter and Chapter 12, Figure 3). Finally, the vagus has general sensory fibers from a small area of the external ear; cell bodies from these are situated in the jugular or superior ganglion.

The motor fibers arise in the nucleus ambiguus of the medulla (Figure 1c and Appendix II, Plate XIV) and leave the brainstem with the parasympathetic fibers. They soon branch away from the vagus and supply all the muscles of the larynx and most of those in the pharynx. Damage to these motor fibers or their nuclei results in a lower motor neuron paralysis, with difficulty in talking (dysphonia) or swallowing (dysphagia).

Note: See Appendix II, Plate XVI for exiting point of cranial nerves.

Chapter 14

The Auditory Pathway

The eighth cranial nerve, the acoustovestibular (vestibulocochlear), is entirely sensory and has two important parts: the acoustic part, which transmits sound impulses from the ear to the brain, and the vestibular part, which is concerned with maintaining body equilibrium. This chapter deals with the acoustic division, which is basically very simple.

In the cochlear apparatus of the inner ear (see Appendix III, Figure 7 and Appendix IV, Figure 5) are situated specialized receptors—the *hair cells*—which are stimulated by auditory vibrations from the external and middle ear. In the cochlea these hair cells synapse with primary neurons, the cell bodies of which are localized in the spiral ganglion, also situated in the cochlea (Figure 1). From here axons pass to the brainstem, enter it at the pontomedullary junction, and immediately bifurcate, with one branch terminating in the *dorsal cochlear nucleus* and the other in the *ventral cochlear nucleus* (Figure 1). From the dorsal cochlear nucleus some secondary axons cross over to the other side and ascend to reach the nucleus of the inferior colliculus. Others do not cross, but ascend ipsilaterally and also terminate in the nucleus of the inferior colliculus (Figure 1). These ascending crossed and uncrossed fibers comprise the *lateral lemniscus.*

Most of the axons from the ventral cochlear nucleus decussate and pass up in the lateral lemniscus to end in the nucleus of the inferior colliculus. A few do not cross over, but ascend in the ipsilateral lateral lemniscus (Figure 1). Thus, both the dorsal and the ventral cochlear nuclei send out crossed and uncrossed fibers to the nucleus of the inferior colliculus. From here fibers are relayed out, via the brachium of the inferior colliculus, to the medial geniculate body, which lies adjacent to the superior colliculus. In this body they synapse with neurons, the axons of which form the auditory radiations that end in the transverse gyri of Heschl located on the dorsomedial surface of the superior temporal gyrus, known as areas 41 and 42—the primary hearing center.

ACCESSORY DETAILS AND CLINICAL ASPECTS

1. The decussating axons from the dorsal and ventral cochlear nuclei form a large distinct mass, the *trapezoid body* (Figure 1).

2. The right and left nuclei of the inferior colliculus are connected to each other by commissural neurons (Figure 1).

3. Some of the fibers in the lateral lemniscus don't end in the nucleus of the inferior colliculus, but pass straight up to the medical geniculate body (Figure 1).

4. On the other hand, many axons from the dorsal and ventral cochlear nuclei do not ascend directly to the midbrain, but rather make many synaptic stops along the way. For example, crossed fibers from both nuclei synapse in the superior olivary nucleus, which then relays up to the higher areas (Figure 1). This is not important clinically. What is important is the fact that each auditory cortex receives fibers from the left and right cochlear nuclei, or put another way, the cochlear nuclei of the right side project onto the left and right auditory cortex, and left cochlear nuclei project to both hearing centers. The clinical significance of this bilateral representation is obvious. If, for example, the right auditory cortex is damaged, then the patient will still hear from both ears, using the intact left auditory cortex. This holds true for damage at other sites along the central pathway; namely, the right medial geniculate body, the right nucleus of the inferior colliculus, or the right lateral lemniscus. However, if the right auditory nerve is cut or damaged anywhere along its path—from the ear up to and including the cochlear nuclei—then the person will be deaf in the right ear, and what holds true for the right side is true for the left.

5. From the nucleus of the inferior colliculus, internuncial axons pass out to various motor centers to mediate auditory reflexes. For example, when one hears a sudden loud noise, the eyes close and the body "jumps," both of which are reactions of the startle reflex.

In the United States, deafness is a widespread problem affecting millions of people. It is generally divided into two main types. The first is *conduction deafness*, or middle ear deafness, in which a mechanical impediment prevents the sound from reaching the cochlea. The impediment may be a torn eardrum, blockage of the auditory canal, or due to other cause. The most common cause, however, is otosclerosis, in which the stapes of the mid-

FIGURE 1

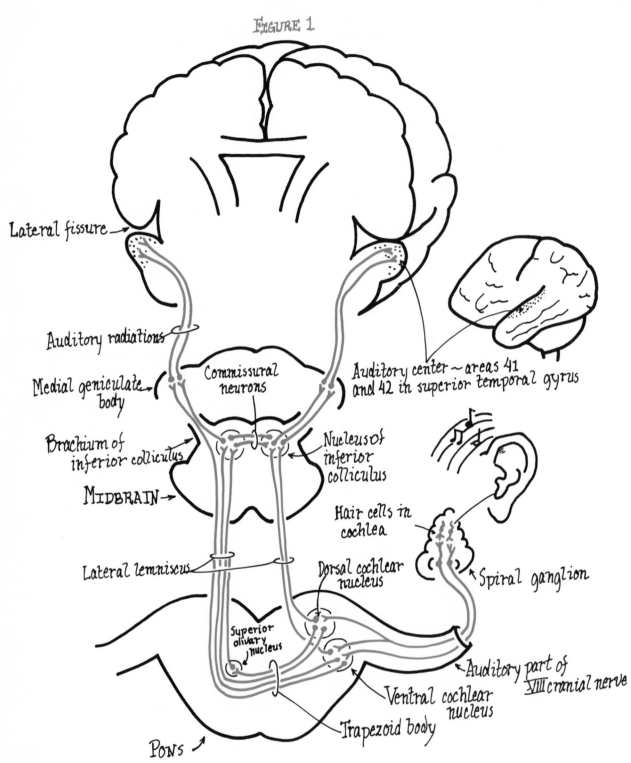

Lateral fissure

Auditory radiations

Medial geniculate body

Commissural neurons

Brachium of inferior colliculus

Nucleus of inferior colliculus

MIDBRAIN→

Auditory center ~ areas 41 and 42 in superior temporal gyrus

Hair cells in cochlea

Spiral ganglion

Lateral lemniscus

Dorsal cochlear nucleus

Superior olivary nucleus

Auditory part of VIII cranial nerve

Ventral cochlear nucleus

Trapezoid body

PONS↗

PLATE 14~1.

dle ear becomes fixed in the cochlea and cannot transmit its vibrations. The second type is *sensorineural deafness*. As its name implies, it is caused by damage to either the cochlea or cranial nerve VIII.

The distinction between these two types is important from both a diagnostic as well as a treatment point of view. In conduction or middle ear deafness, a patient will hear poorly or not at all a vibrating tuning fork that is placed near the ear. However, the patient will hear the tuning fork if it is placed against the skull, because now the vibrations bypass the middle ear and are transmitted directly to the cochlea. On the other hand, in sensorineural deafness the patient will have difficulty in hearing a vibrating tuning fork both via air conduction and via bone conduction.

In recent years great progress has been made in the treatment of middle ear deafness, especially in otosclerosis. By means of microsurgery, the fixed stapes can be made mobile or even replaced, and the majority of patients show great improvement in their hearing.

There are many causes for sensorineural deafness, but the list below mentions only the most common:

1. Rubella infection in a pregnant woman very often causes her child to be born totally deaf.
2. Some antibiotics (e.g., streptomycin and neomycin) when given in large doses may cause partial or total deafness, often accompanied by vestibular disturbances.
3. Atrophy of the cochlea is one of the most common causes of deafness in the aged.
4. Such tumors as acoustic neuroma of cranial nerve VIII can produce deafness.
5. There are many forms of hereditary deafness based on genetic defects.

In sensorineural deafness, doctors can now implant a wire with the electrodes inserted into the cochlea. The other end of the special wire ends at the surface of the skull. There it is attached to a wire from a microphone-sound processor which picks up and converts sound waves into electrical impulses. Thus the auditory nerve is stimulated.

Chapter 15

Visual Pathways
and Optic Reflexes

The visual pathways are among the more important pathways of the nervous system. Because injuries to them are common, the physician must know and understand them "cold."

Light rays from an object in the visual field enter the eyeball (Appendix III, Figure 6), are inverted by the lens, and strike the nervous layer, the *retina.* The retina is composed of several layers and types of neurons, among them being the light-sensitive *rods* and *cones.* Each eye has a temporal and a nasal visual field, and because of the inversion by the lens, the temporal visual field is projected onto the nasal retinal field and the nasal visual field falls on the temporal retinal field (Figure 1). Loss of vision is always described with reference to the visual fields, not the retinal fields. These concepts can be quite confusing at first, and it pays the student to read and review each concept slowly and attentively.

Axons from nerve cells in the eye pass posteriorly in the optic nerve (Appendix III, Figure 6). At the chiasma, those from the nasal retinal field cross over to join the axons from the temporal retinal field, which do not cross (Figure 1). Together they continue posteriorly in the optic tract and end in the lateral geniculate body of the diencephalon. Here they synapse with neurons that sweep out to form the optic radiations, which end in the visual cortex of the occipital lobe. This cortex begins at the occipital pole and is situated on the *cuneate* and *lingual gyri,* which border on the *calcarine fissure* (Figures 1 and 2). Thus, the left visual field of each eye is represented on the right occipital cortex, whereas the right visual fields are represented on the left occipital cortex (Figure 1). The lens also inverts the upper visual field onto the lower part of the retina and vice versa (Figure 2). This pattern is maintained throughout the pathway, so that the cuneate gyrus, which is above the calcarine fissure, receives impulses from the lower visual field, and the lingual gyrus, which is below the fissure, gets impulses from the upper visual field (Figure 2). Finally, the *macula*—the central area of the retina where vision is the sharpest—sends its impulses to the occipital poles (Figure 1).

CLINICAL ASPECTS

In an eye examination, the fields of vision of each eye are tested and mapped out. If, for example, the right optic nerve is damaged (Example 1, Figure 1) both fields of vision of that eye are affected—in short, *anopsia* or *blindness* of the right eye results.

Example 2 in Figure 1 illustrates how an *aneurysm* of the right internal carotid artery, which lies adjacent to the lateral part of the optic chiasma, can interfere with the temporal axons from the right retina, thus producing *hemianopsia* (half-blindness) in the right eye. Because the visual field affected is the nasal field, we speak of a nasal hemianopsia of the right eye, or right nasal hemianopsia.

Example 3 in Figure 1 shows how the pituitary gland, lying below the optic tracts near the chiasma, can develop an expanding tumor that presses on the decussating nasal axons. This can produce hemianopsia in the temporal visual field of both eyes—a *bitemporal hemianopsia.*

Examples 4, 5, and 6 in Figure 1 illustrate how a lesion in the right optic tract, the right optic radiations, or the right visual cortex can produce loss of vision in the left visual fields of both eyes, which is called a *left homonymous hemianopsia.*

Because the visual field of each eye is divided into nasal and temporal parts plus upper and lower parts, the term "quadrant" is used to denote them (e.g., upper quadrant or lower right quadrant). There can also be various quadrantic anopsias.

OPTIC REFLEXES

If light from a small source, such as a pencil flashlight, is shone into one eye from a short distance, there will be pupillary reflex constriction in both eyes—a reaction known as a *consensual reflex.* As you have just learned, optic tract fibers end in the lateral geniculate body. However, about 1% of them peel off just before reaching the geniculate body and terminate in the pretectal nucleus of the midbrain (Figure 3). From here internuncial fibers pass to the parasympathetic Edinger-Westphal nucleus,

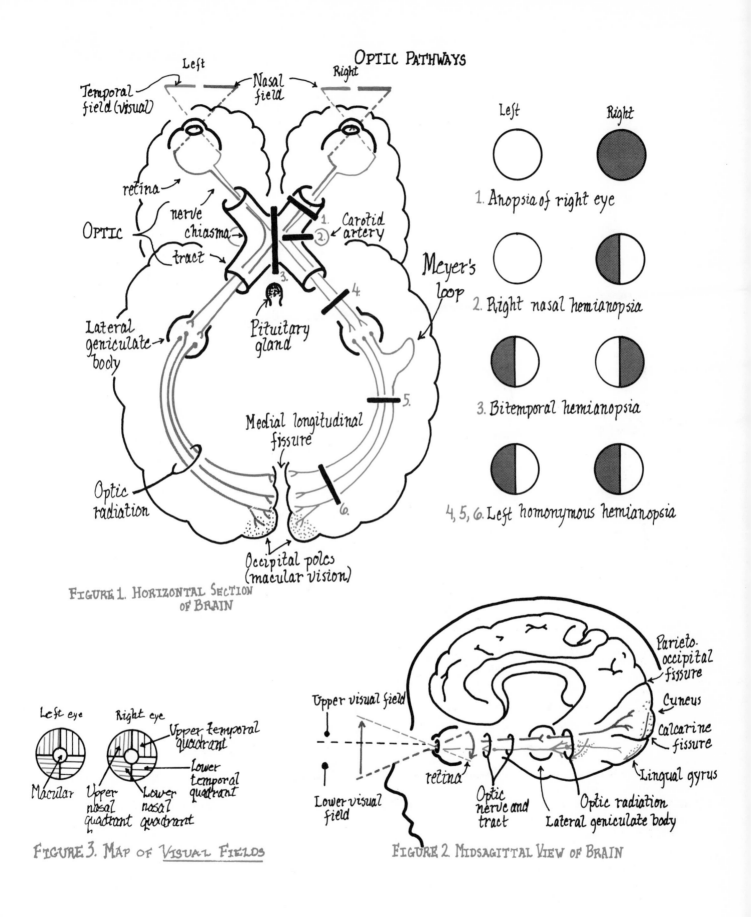

OPTIC PATHWAYS

Left   Nasal   Right

Temporal field (visual)

Nasal field

retina

OPTIC   nerve

chiasma

tract

Carotid artery

1.

2.

3.

Meyer's loop

Lateral geniculate body

Pituitary gland

4.

Medial longitudinal fissure

5.

Optic radiation

6.

Occipital poles (macular vision)

FIGURE 1. HORIZONTAL SECTION OF BRAIN

Left   Right

1. Anopsia of right eye

2. Right nasal hemianopsia

3. Bitemporal hemianopsia

4, 5, 6. Left homonymous hemianopsia

Left eye   Right eye

Upper temporal quadrant

Lower temporal quadrant

Macular   Upper nasal quadrant   Lower nasal quadrant

FIGURE 3. MAP OF VISUAL FIELDS

Upper visual field

Lower visual field

retina

Optic nerve and tract

Parieto-occipital fissure

Cuneus

Calcarine fissure

Lingual gyrus

Optic radiation

Lateral geniculate body

FIGURE 2. MIDSAGITTAL VIEW OF BRAIN

PLATE 15~1.

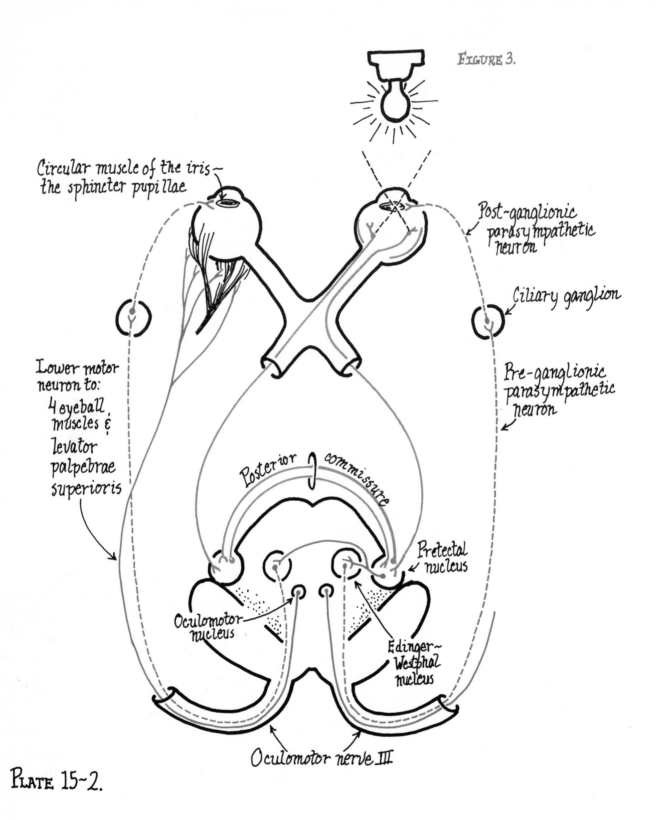

FIGURE 3.

Circular muscle of the iris ~
the sphincter pupillae

Post-ganglionic
parasympathetic
neuron

Ciliary ganglion

Lower motor
neuron to:
4 eyeball
muscles &
levator
palpebrae
superioris

Pre-ganglionic
parasympathetic
neuron

Posterior commissure

Pretectal
nucleus

Oculomotor
nucleus

Edinger~
Westphal
nucleus

Oculomotor nerve III

PLATE 15~2.

which then automatically discharges motor stimuli to the circular muscle of the iris, causing pupillary constriction (Figure 3). Therefore, there are three ways that light impulses from one eye can cause reflex constriction in both pupils:

1. Some optic fibers from the right eye's nasal retinal field cross in the chiasma to reach the contralateral pretectal nucleus (Figure 3).
2. The right and left pretectal nuclei are interconnected by commissural neurons that pass through the posterior commissure. Therefore, a stimulus reaching one nucleus is relayed to the other (Figure 3).
3. Each pretectal nucleus sends out fibers to both the right and left Edinger-Westphal nucleus (Figure 3).

CLINICAL ASPECTS

The pupillary light reflex is one of the most useful and important reflexes in medical practice. It occurs even when a person is unconscious. If it cannot be elicited, a serious condition in the CNS, especially the brainstem, is indicated.

In a person who is dying the pupils often dilate markedly and do not contract to light. On the other hand, in persons who have taken such narcotics as heroin or morphine the pupils constrict greatly ("pinpoint pupils") and do not dilate. This fact is often used by police officers and physicians to determine whether a person is intoxicated on such drugs.

Pupillary reflexes—dilation (mydriasis) and/or constriction (myosis)—are also very important in general anesthesia. Here, according to the degree of dilation or constriction (as well as other signs), the anesthetist knows very accurately what stages and planes the patient is in. (Stages and planes refer to the degrees of depth of unconsciousness.)

The Edinger-Westphal nucleus is also concerned with the accommodation reflex, whereby the lens of the eye accommodates itself for near and far vision. From this nucleus, motor stimuli are sent out over the pre- and postganglionic fibers to reach the ciliary muscle that controls the anteroposterior (front-to-back) diameter of the lens. This is a complex reflex that involves cortical areas, as well as the *nucleus of Perla*, which is concerned with the convergence of the eyes.

In Chapter 12 it was mentioned that doctors often put an atropine solution in the eye to dilate the pupil and so have a larger "window" to look through.* However one must first make sure that the patient doesn't have glaucoma because dilation in these patients can bring a rapid, sharp increase in the intraocular pressure with damage to the sensitive retina.

Glaucoma is a group of acute or chronic diseases of the eye, where the intraocular pressure rises above 29 mm Hg; if left untreated it can result in blindness. (Even with detection and treatment it is a major cause of blindness in the United States). A frequent pathognomonic sign is the patient's complaint of seeing haloes around light sources. However not all patients experience this phenomenon, and some do not even know that they have the disease. Therefore one tests for glaucoma by having the patient lie down, and by placing a tonometer on the corneal surface one easily obtains a reading of the intraocular pressure, which normally ranges between 13–29 mm Hg.

---

*Today better drugs than atropine, which causes prolonged accommodation paralysis, are available.

The Olfactory System

Many lower animal forms, such as dogs, deer, amphibians, and certain birds, depend primarily on the sense of smell to locate food, to distinguish friend from foe, and to attract the opposite sex. Consequently, the olfactory system is very highly developed in these animals and is closely connected to the aggressive drive, because this drive is necessary to obtain the above-mentioned objects. In humans, the sense of smell is probably the least important of the major senses, but its pathways, carried over from lower forms, are the most complex of the nervous system. Furthermore, there are a great deal of contradictory data, based on experiments in animals, and beginning students who open most neuroanatomy texts find themselves immersed in a welter of conflicting theories couched in the most obtuse and strange terminology. (It is a rule of thumb in science, medicine, and other subjects that the more theories and the more terminology there are concerning a subject, the less is known about it; psychology, psychoanalysis, and economics are excellent examples of this.) This chapter discusses the basic, generally agreed-upon facts concerning the olfactory system and touches very lightly on the experimental data.

In the epithelial tissue of the nasal cavity are located receptor cells sensitive to smell. These first-order neurons, which are bipolar, pass up into the olfactory bulb, where they synapse with second-order neurons whose axons form the olfactory tract. This tract runs posteriorly and then bifurcates into lateral and medial olfactory tracts, or *stria* (Figures 1 and 2). The area between the bifurcating stria forms the anterior perforated area (Figure 2). The axons of the medial olfactory stria terminate in the paraolfactory (septal) area and the anterior perforated area, while some enter the anterior commissure and cross over to terminate in the contralateral septal area (Figures 1 and 2). The fibers of the lateral olfactory stria end in the cortex of the uncus and in the underlying amygdaloid nucleus (Figures 1 and 2). It is believed that the septal area, the anterior perforated substance, and the cortex of the uncus are the cerebral areas concerned with the "interpretation" of smell (i.e., the primary olfactory areas or centers).

In humans the sense of smell can trigger memories, various emotions, and their related reflexes. For example, the smell of good food causes pleasure and salivation, whereas that of rotten eggs causes disgust, nausea, and even vomiting. An enticing perfume may result in sexual arousal (isn't that its basic purpose?), whereas other odors may elicit long-forgotten memories.

The major reflex pathways are as follows: From the amygdaloid nucleus, fibers collect in a bundle, the *stria terminalis*, which loops around and terminates in the hypothalamus (Figure 3). The amygdala also sends short fibers to the adjacent hippocampus, where they synapse with neurons that form a large bundle, the *fornix*. This distinctive tract curves up and around to end in the mammillary bodies of the hypothalamus (Figure 3). Finally, from the septal or paraolfactory area, short fibers pass to terminate also in the hypothalamus (Figure 3). It isn't surprising that all these reflex pathways end in the hypothalamus, for, as shown in the following chapter, this is the main coordination and reflex-discharge center for many sensations, such as smell, taste, and emotions, as well as being the control center of the autonomic nervous system. Reflex-discharge pathways carry smell sensations from the hypothalamus to the appropriate motor nuclei and reticular areas in the brainstem. The two main tracts are the mamillotegmental and the dorsal longitudinal fasciculus (Figure 3). Finally, from the mammillary bodies there is a large bundle, the mamillothalamic tract, which ends in the anterior group of the thalamic nuclei. From here the impulses are relayed to the cingulate gyrus (Figure 3). In spite of much experimental work, no functional significance of this pathway has been discovered.

ACCESSORY DETAILS

The limbic system refers to the numerous olfactory reflex centers and their various pathways. These include the amygdala, hippocampus, pyriform area, fornix, stria terminalis, stria medullaris thalmae, indusium griseum, median forebrain bundle, habenula, habenular commissure, fasciculus retroflexus, diagonal band of Broca, etc. All this may be interesting from a theoretical point of view and for those doing experimental research, but there is no "rhyme or reason" why medical students should be required to know these complicated pathways and connections.

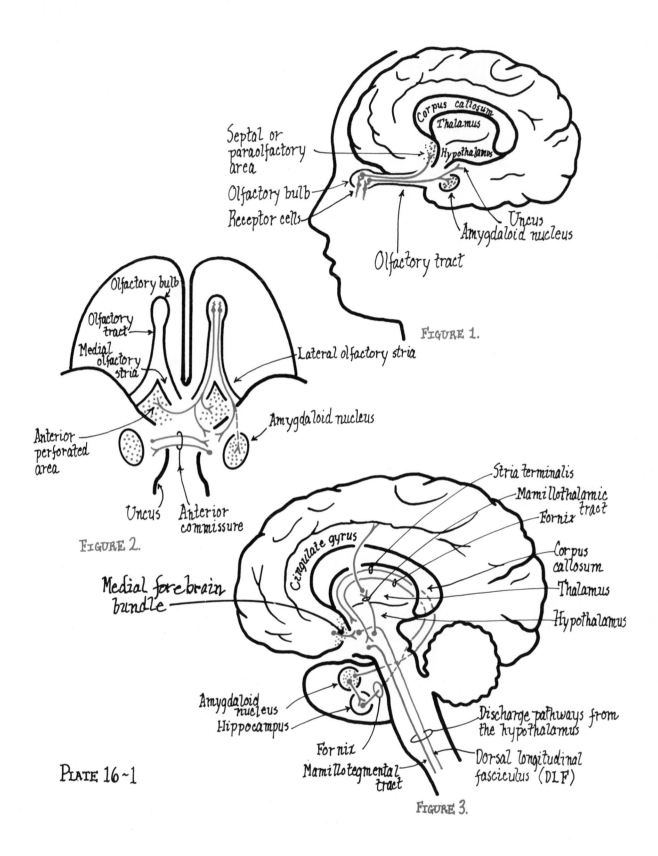

Septal or paraolfactory area

Olfactory bulb

Receptor cells

Corpus callosum

Thalamus

Hypothalamus

Uncus

Amygdaloid nucleus

Olfactory tract

FIGURE 1.

Olfactory bulb

Olfactory tract

Medial olfactory stria

Lateral olfactory stria

Anterior perforated area

Amygdaloid nucleus

Uncus

Anterior commissure

FIGURE 2.

Cingulate gyrus

Stria terminalis

Mamillothalamic tract

Fornix

Corpus callosum

Thalamus

Hypothalamus

Medial forebrain bundle

Amygdaloid nucleus

Hippocampus

Fornix

Mamillotegmental tract

Discharge pathways from the hypothalamus

Dorsal longitudinal fasciculus (DLF)

FIGURE 3.

PLATE 16~1

59

CLINICAL ASPECTS

Loss of smell results from damage to the receptor cells, the olfactory bulb, or the olfactory tract and is known medically as *anosmia*. Lesions of the temporal lobe in the area of the uncus and the amygdala often produce olfactory hallucinations, epileptic seizures, or a combination of both, known as *uncinate fits* when the epileptic fit is preceded by an olfactory aura that has an unpleasant smell.

In monkeys the removal of the amygdala results in very docile, somnolent animals, whereas in cats the same procedure produces animals who are very aggressive in unprovoked situations—a condition known as sham rage. However, in both species the procedure causes a greatly increased sexual drive.

DIAGNOSTIC TESTS

The sense of smell is tested separately in each nostril. Close one nostril and then pass, successively, vials containing various nonirritative substances, such as pine oil, coffee, and perfume under the open nostril. Ask the patient if he or she smells the substance and can identify it. A gradual unilateral loss of smell may indicate the presence of a tumor in the frontal lobe.

A good sense of smell is also a useful diagnostic tool for the physician or paramedic. For example, the underlying cause of a patient's coma may be deduced by the odor of the breath. In diabetic coma the breath smells like sweet-spoiled fruit. Alcohol has its own well-known smell (vodka being excepted), whereas uremic coma produces a uriniferous odor. In hepatic coma there is a stinking musty smell to the breath.

Chapter 17

The Reticular System

The reticular system is a phylogenetically old system that is divided anatomically and physiologically into two parts—a descending and an ascending formation.

DESCENDING RETICULAR FORMATION

The descending reticular formation is a system concerned with:

1. Relaying impulses from the hypothalamus to various target organs of the autonomic nervous system
2. Relaying involuntary motor impulses from the extrapyramidal systems to voluntary muscles.

Scattered deep in the brainstem are the groups of diffuse nuclei or areas (some authors and investigators call them "formations") belonging to this system. In the midbrain they are called the *deep* and *dorsal tegmental nuclei*, in the pons they are called the *central tegmental nucleus*, and in the medulla they are the *central* and *inferior nuclei*. Some books also mention other descending reticular nuclei or call them by different names, but the main point to grasp is not the exact number of nuclei but the fact that they exist and their function.

These nuclei or formations receive stimuli from the hypothalamus fiber tracts, such as the dorsal longitudinal fasciculus and the mamillotegmental tract (Figure 1). In addition, various basal ganglia, such as the globus pallidus, the substantia nigra, and the subthalamic nucleus, project fibers that terminate in these nuclei. Lastly, the vestibular system, which is also extrapyramidal, sends some of its fibers to the reticular nuclei (see Chapters 10 and 11).

These incoming fibers synapse with neurons whose axons then leave the reticular nuclei and form the lateral and medial reticulospinal tracts. These are descending, crossed, and uncrossed, multisynaptic pathways that travel down to all levels of the spinal cord in the lateral and ventral white columns. In the cord they synapse either on the ventral horn cells, which form the final common pathway, or on the preganglionic neurons in the intermediate gray horn.

ASCENDING RETICULAR FORMATION

The ascending reticular formation, better known as the reticular activating system, is concerned with degrees of conscious alertness, as well as with sleep. Situated in the medulla, pons, and midbrain are groups of poorly defined nuclei connected to each other by a chain of multisynaptic neurons. Because the nuclei and their interconnecting chain have a diffuse and poorly defined appearance, they were given the name *reticular system.*

All the major sensory pathways (e.g., the spinothalamic, for pain, temperature, touch, and pressure; the auditory; the visual) send collateral axons that end in the nuclei of the reticular activating system. These nuclei then send the sensory stimuli they have received up the multisynaptic chain, which ends primarily in a group of nuclei of the thalamus known as the midline group. As has already been shown, the thalamus serves as a relay center for many sensory pathways, as well as motor ones, and it is not surprising that it also serves as a relay for the reticular activating system. From the thalamic midline, nuclei impulses are relayed up to the cerebral cortex, where they influence states of mental alertness and sleep. Exactly how these impulses are relayed and what specific regions of the cerebral cortex they reach are not known.

Sleeping animals and humans exhibit a characteristic electroencephalogram (EEG) wave pattern, but if the reticular activating nuclei of sleeping animals are experimentally stimulated, the animals awaken, and we see that the change from sleep to wakefulness is accompanied by a change in the EEG wave pattern. In animals that are already awake, stimulation of the reticular activating nuclei produces states of greater alertness accompanied by characteristic changes in the EEG pattern. It is therefore assumed that alertness and/or sleep is largely dependent on the amount of stimuli reaching the cerebral cortex via the reticular activating system. If the amount of stimuli from the outside world is reduced, there will be a lowering of alertness, and sleep may result. On the other hand, an increase in the amount of stimulation reaching the cerebral cortex via the ascending reticular for-

FIGURE 1. SCHEMATIC DIAGRAM OF THE DESCENDING RETICULAR FORMATION

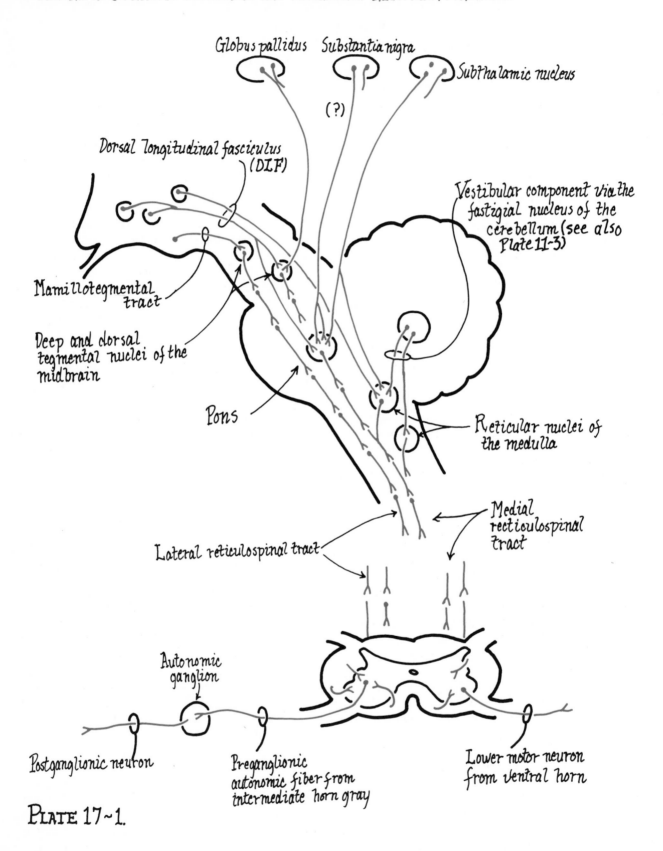

Globus pallidus   Substantia nigra

Subthalamic nucleus

(?)

Dorsal longitudinal fasciculus (DLF)

Vestibular component via the fastigial nucleus of the cerebellum (see also Plate 11-3)

Mamillotegmental tract

Deep and dorsal tegmental nuclei of the midbrain

Pons

Reticular nuclei of the medulla

Medial reticulospinal tract

Lateral reticulospinal tract

Autonomic ganglion

Postganglionic neuron

Preganglionic autonomic fiber from intermediate horn gray

Lower motor neuron from ventral horn

PLATE 17~1.

mation results in greater alertness. In a nutshell, we may say that:

↓stimulation from various sensory systems into the reticular nuclei → ↓ amount of stimulation to the thalamic midline nuclei → ↓ stimulus to cerebral cortex → ↓ altertness and/or sleep

This simple outline is just one aspect of an extremely complex picture, most of which is still unknown to us. One should not conclude that sleep or alertness is totally dependent on the state of the reticular activating system; there are many other factors (e.g., metabolic and psychological factors) that play a part in alertness and sleep. This is especially important as one of the first questions asked by a physician who is trying to determine a patient's general status is: "How are you sleeping and eating?" There are also many factors that we know nothing about, the discovery of which will throw new light on the problem of sleep, alertness, and consciousness.

CLINICAL ASPECTS

Although there is no known center for sleep or consciousness, it is believed that the reticular formation in the brainstem is primarily involved because damage to it often produces states of unconsciousness or coma. (This is known by postmortem examination of the brain.) The author has a friend who was sitting in a car that had stopped for a red light. It was struck from behind by another car, and the driver suffered a severe whiplash—with no other known injuries—and has been in a coma for over 2 years.

Concussion

This is usually defined as a transient state of unconsciousness caused by a sudden sharp blow to the head. Upon awakening there may be episodes of vomiting.

Stupor

This is a state of unconsciousness from which the patient is aroused with difficulty and when awake is mentally confused.

Coma

This is a state of unconsciousness resembling sleep from which the individual cannot be roused even by the strongest stimuli. Coma varies in degree. For example, in deep coma there is a complete absence of response to stimuli, and most reflexes are lost. In lighter stages the patient may respond to sounds, some reflexes and movements are present, and the eyes may be open. Many pathologic conditions can produce coma or comatose states, but the three most common causes are alcoholism or other drug intoxications, injuries to the head, and cerebrovascular accidents (CVAs; strokes).

From a diagnostic perspective the etiology of coma falls into three main groups:

1. *Structural: Trauma and CVA*
   Pupillary reflexes nearly always absent; intracranial pressure is increased; EEG normal.
2. *Toxic: Alcohol, drugs, or poisons*
   Pupillary reflexes nearly always present; no increase in intracranial pressure; EEG normal.
3. *Metabolic: Diabetic acidosis, hypoglycemia, hepatic problems, Addisonian crises, etc.*
   Pupillary reflexes nearly always present; no increase in cerebrospinal fluid (CSF) pressure; *EEG nearly always abnormal*. (Remember that your sense of smell can help you deduct the cause—see diagnostic tests in preceding chapter.)

From a treatment point of view, remember to do ABCD.

A—Maintain *airway and avoid aspiration* by correct positioning of patient.

B—Maintain and monitor *blood pressure*.

C—Avoid cardiac and *circulatory collapse*.

D—Start making *diagnosis and draw* blood for chemical analysis.

Chapter 18

The Hypothalamus

The hypothalamus is one of the smallest areas of the brain, yet no other region has so many different and vital functions. As its name indicates, it lies beneath the thalamus. It is seen well in a midsagittal section (Plates III and IV in Appendix II), where it extends from the lamina terminalis to the midbrain. Separating it from the overlying thalamus is a shallow groove, the *hypothalamic sulcus.* The hypothalamus thus forms the lateral wall of the lower part of the third ventricle and is also seen in cross-sections (Plate VII in Appendix II). If one looks at the base of the brain, the hypothalamus is seen as forming the area that lies posterior to the optic chiasma and includes the infundibulum and mammillary bodies. Packed into this small region are many nuclei and areas (Figure 1) that are concerned with such functions as temperature control, sleep, water metabolism, secretion of hormones, control of blood pressure, hunger, and maintenance of balance between the sympathetic and parasympathetic divisions. It also plays a part in emotional reactions and possibly other situations.

HEAT REGULATION

The anterior hypothalamic area is concerned with heat regulation of the body. When there is an increase in body temperature, the heated blood passes through the anterior hypothalamic area and sets off a mechanism that facilitates heat loss (Figure 2). Fibers leave the anterior hypothalamic area and join the dorsal longitudinal fasciculus (DLF), which is the major descending pathway from the hypothalamus. The DLF terminates in the descending reticular nuclei of the brainstem, where it synapses with neurons of the medial and lateral reticulospinal tracts. These then descend the cord and stimulate the sympathetic nervous system and voluntary muscles. Other fibers of the DLF terminate in and stimulate the cardiac and respiratory centers in the medulla. The results of all these stimuli are the following reactions, which serve to reduce body temperature:

1. Dilation of peripheral blood vessels beneath the skin, with a subsequent increase in heat radiation.
2. An increase in sweating, which reduces heat. (Evaporation is a cooling process.)

3. Increase in respiratory rate, with "blowing off" of hot air from the lungs.
4. A decrease in the body's metabolic rate.
5. Increases in peripheral blood flow accompanied by increased heat dissipation.

If we experimentally destroy an animal's anterior hypothalamic region, it becomes unable to respond to heat increases in its environment. Thus, when the temperature rises, its body temperature rises, and eventually it will die from heat prostration.

Cold regulation is controlled by the posterior hypothalamic area. When the temperature of the environment drops, the body becomes cooler. The cooled blood passes through the posterior hypothalamic area (Figure 2) and sets off a mechanism that is directly the opposite of the one just discussed. The pathways are basically the same—the DLF, reticular nuclei, and reticulospinal tracts. The reactions set off to conserve body heat are as follows:

1. Peripheral vasoconstriction, with a subsequent decrease in the amount of heat lost by radiation
2. A decrease in peripheral blood flow
3. An increase in body metabolism
4. Shivering of voluntary muscles. Shivering is work in which energy, in the form of heat, is produced. (There is, of course, also energy of motion.)
5. A decrease in the respiratory rate.

Experimental lesions in the posterior hypothalamic area of animals prevent them from adjusting to cold environments, and their bodies become as cold as the surroundings.

WATER BALANCE (OSMOREGULATION)

The hypothalamic mechanism for maintaining water balance is one of the most interesting regulatory mechanisms of the body. It is known that a hormone from the posterior pituitary body, called antidiuretic hormone or ADH, acts on the distal convoluted tubules of the kidney, causing resorption of water. If the amount of ADH produced is reduced, a pathologic condition known as diabetes insipidus results. In this disease the patient urinates 18–20 liters of urine per day instead of the normal 1–2 liters and also drinks large amounts of fluids (polydipsia) to replace those lost. The regula-

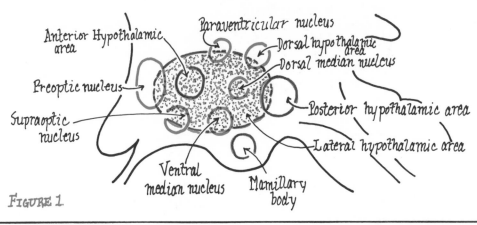

Anterior Hypothalamic area

Paraventricular nucleus

Dorsal hypothalamic area

Dorsal median nucleus

Preoptic nucleus

Supraoptic nucleus

Posterior hypothalamic area

Lateral hypothalamic area

Ventral median nucleus

Mamillary body

FIGURE 1.

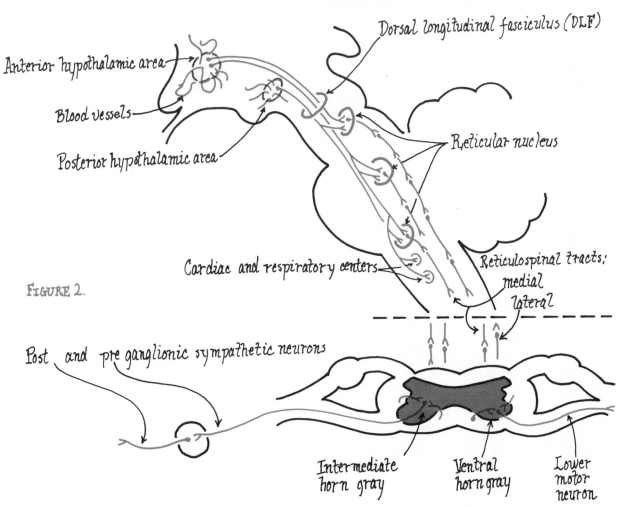

Dorsal longitudinal fasciculus (DLF)

Anterior hypothalamic area

Blood vessels

Posterior hypothalamic area

Reticular nucleus

Cardiac and respiratory centers

Reticulospinal tracts; medial lateral

FIGURE 2.

Post and pre ganglionic sympathetic neurons

Intermediate horn gray

Ventral horn gray

Lower motor neuron

PLATE 18-1.

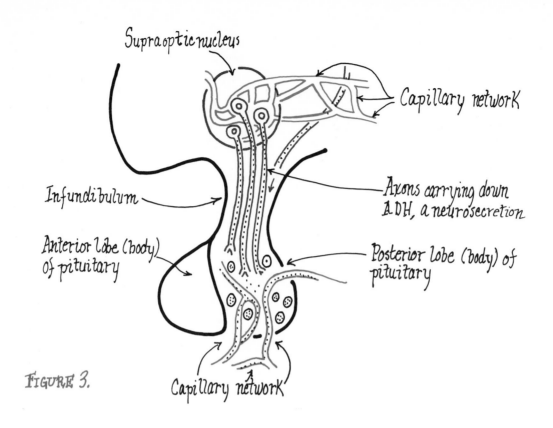

Supraoptic nucleus

Capillary network

Infundibulum

Axons carrying down
A.D.H, a neurosecretion

Anterior lobe (body)
of pituitary

Posterior lobe (body) of
pituitary

FIGURE 3.

Capillary network

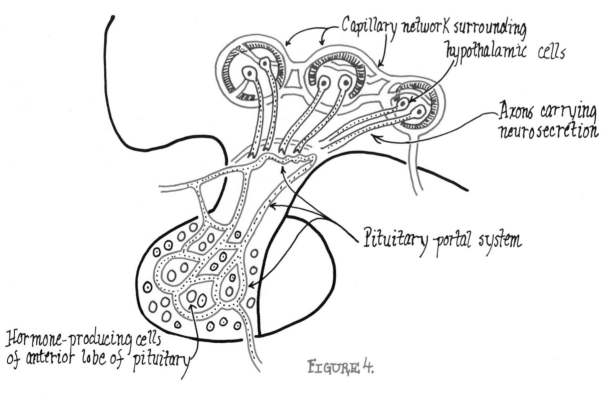

Capillary network surrounding
hypothalamic cells

Axons carrying
neurosecretion

Pituitary portal system

Hormone-producing cells
of anterior lobe of pituitary

FIGURE 4.

PLATE 18~2.

tory mechanism in the production and release of ADH is a function of the supraoptic nucleus of the hypothalamus. The cells of this nucleus and possibly those of the paraventricular nucleus produce ADH, and this neurosecretion passes down the axons of the neurons, via the infundibulum, to reach the cells of the posterior pituitary (Figure 3), where the ADH is either stored or released into the capillary network.

If there is a reduction in the amount of water in the blood, the cells of the supraoptic nucleus, which are sensitive to such a change, will produce and release more ADH. This results in more water being resorbed by the kidney tubules and its conservation by the body. On the other hand, if there is a state of hydration, the cells of the supraoptic nucleus react by decreasing the production and release of ADH. This decrease in the production and release of ADH results in a decrease in the amount of water resorption by the kidneys, and therefore a greater amount is urinated (polyuria).

INFLUENCE OF THE HYPOTHALAMUS ON THE SECRETION OF HORMONES FROM THE ANTERIOR LOBE OF THE PITUITARY

There is much evidence that cells of the hypothalamus *can in part* influence the secretion of various hormones of the anterior lobe of the pituitary gland. The mechanism resembles that of water metabolism. Neurosecretory cells of the hypothalamus are very sensitive to the blood concentration of the various anterior lobe hormones. In response to a decrease, these neurons produce a neurosecretion that passes down the axons. However, the axons terminate in the region of the infundibulum, and here the neurosecretion is "picked up" by a pituitary portal system (Figure 4). This carries the neurosecretion to the anterior lobe, where it stimulates the cells to produce the various hormones. One must not conclude that the hypothalamus is the only, or principal, regulator of hormones from the anterior lobe. There are other mechanisms, such as a direct feedback control, as well as mechanisms that are not yet clearly understood.

HYPOTHALAMIC DISCHARGE IN EMOTIONAL STATES

Various emotional states, such as anger, fear, or well-being, result in physiologic reactions. The hy-pothalamus is a center for the control and discharge of such reactions. For example, when one sees or hears something that evokes an angry reaction, the stimuli first reach various areas of the cerebral cortex, such as the visual or auditory centers, the memory centers, or the personality area of the frontal lobe, all of which are interconnected by association tracts. From the cerebral cortex, especially its frontal lobe, there is a discharge pathway to the hypothalamus. From the latter, the major descending pathway is the dorsal longitudinal fasciculus, which arises from all the hypothalamic nuclei and areas except the supraoptic and ventral median nucleus. (A minor pathway is the mamillotegmental tract.) The dorsal longitudinal fasciculus leaves the hypothalamus and passes down the length of the brainstem, where it gives off branches to all the descending reticular nuclei; all the parasympathetic nuclei of cranial nerves III, VII, IX, and X; the respiratory and cardiac centers; and the motor nuclei of the cranial nerves (Figure 2). From the reticular nuclei emerge the lateral and medial reticulospinal tracts, which descend the cord to supply the autonomic nervous system, as well as the voluntary muscles. Thus, we see the complex interrelationship that exists among various parts of the brain, and one must proceed with great caution in applying new surgical or other techniques, such as lobotomies.

The hypothalamus is also involved in the olfactory reflex system (see Chapter 16). Finally, experimental work in animals has demonstrated that destruction of the ventral median nucleus produces animals with voracious, almost insatiable, appetites, whereas destruction of the lateral hypothalamic area produces animals that have no appetite. Clinically, we see that some patients who have tumors of the hypothalamus lose their appetites and become emaciated.

CLINICAL ASPECTS

Many weight-reducing compounds contain substances that inhibit the appetite centers. This action results in decreased appetite—and, it is hoped, reduced weight.

Chapter 19

The Cerebral Cortex

The cerebral cortex is most highly developed in humans. It is responsible for the qualities that distinguish humans from other animals—for example, the ability to use the hand for skilled and intricate movements, a very high level of speech, symbolic thought, personality, and conscience. We know all this because if certain areas of the cortex are damaged these qualities are lost or greatly reduced.

In submammalian species the cerebral cortex is small and concerned almost exclusively with smell, which, as has already been described, is for them one of the most important sensations. The thalamus is the main sensory receptor area, and the basal ganglia and subthalamic nuclei serve as the motor discharge areas. Because fine, complicated, voluntary movements are not seen in these lower forms, the cerebellum is primarily a center for equilibrium, which is a function of its flocculonodular lobe. As one ascends the evolutionary ladder, the cerebral cortex enlarges and takes on other functions. For example, the main sensory area is now localized in the postcentral gyrus, and its former center, the thalamus, now becomes a center that relays the sensory impulses from the body to the cortex. With the appearance of the cerebral motor cortex, the basal ganglia in humans become areas of crude motor activity. Parallel with the development of this motor cortex there is a great development of the cerebellum as a coordination center for muscle activity, but the floccular nodulus remains the center for body equilibrium. In humans some functions, such as smell, decrease greatly in importance, although the complicated pathways remain—and drive medical students up the walls.

With the increase in complexity and functions there is an increase in the number of neurons, and the area of cerebral cortex increases to such a degree that the cortex, in order to expand in the same volume area, is thrown into folds, giving the characteristic appearance of gyri and sulci (see Appendix III, Figures 1–5). (In lower forms, such as the rat, the surface of the cerebral cortex is smooth.) This same principle is used by restaurant owners in high-rent areas—instead of having straight counters they make them convoluted and thus squeeze in more customers.

As has been mentioned throughout this text, certain areas of the cortex have specific functions. The precentral gyrus (area 4) is concerned with initiating voluntary movements, whereas the post-central gyrus (area 3, 1, 2) is the primary somatic sensory reception center. The occipital pole and the area on both sides of the calcarine fissure (area 17) form the primary visual receptor center. Areas 41 and 42, Heschls gyri, situated on the superior temporal gyrus, are the primary auditory reception center. Damage to any of these areas results in a loss of function, such as paralysis, anesthesia, or blindness. In addition, area 8, lying anterior to area 6 in the frontal lobe (Figure 1), is concerned with voluntary conjugate movements of the eyes. The frontal poles and the areas surrounding them are the site of personality. A person who suffers injury to this area—say, following a car accident—will probably undergo personality changes. The author remembers a case of a very friendly and pleasant social worker who suddenly and for no apparent reason became very argumentative and abusive, until her death a short while later. Autopsy revealed an expanding tumor in the frontal lobe that had caused both her death and the marked changes in character.

In the mid-1930s a Portuguese neurosurgeon, Moniz, introduced the procedure of cutting or removing parts of the frontal lobes—a lobotomy—as a means of treating severely psychotic patients. With hardly a murmur of dissent, this procedure was widely hailed (Moniz received the Nobel prize for it in 1949) and widely practiced. True, after the operation many of the patients were quieter and more docile, but they also lost all initiative, became indifferent to their surroundings, defecated and urinated in public, and showed other behavioral disturbances. Today this barbarous operation is thoroughly discredited. Any surgeon contemplating it should take into account, among other things, the fact that Moniz was almost murdered by a former patient who was distraught over his new state. This was one case where the operation was a success, but the surgeon nearly died!

Surrounding each of the primary cortical areas and closely allied with them are *associated areas*. Around the visual area (area 17) there are areas 18 and 19, which have several functions. First, they are concerned with "interpreting" the visual impulses that reach area 17. We see round, red objects in front of us, and areas 18 and 19 interpret them as apples. This interpretation is called *gnosis*, from

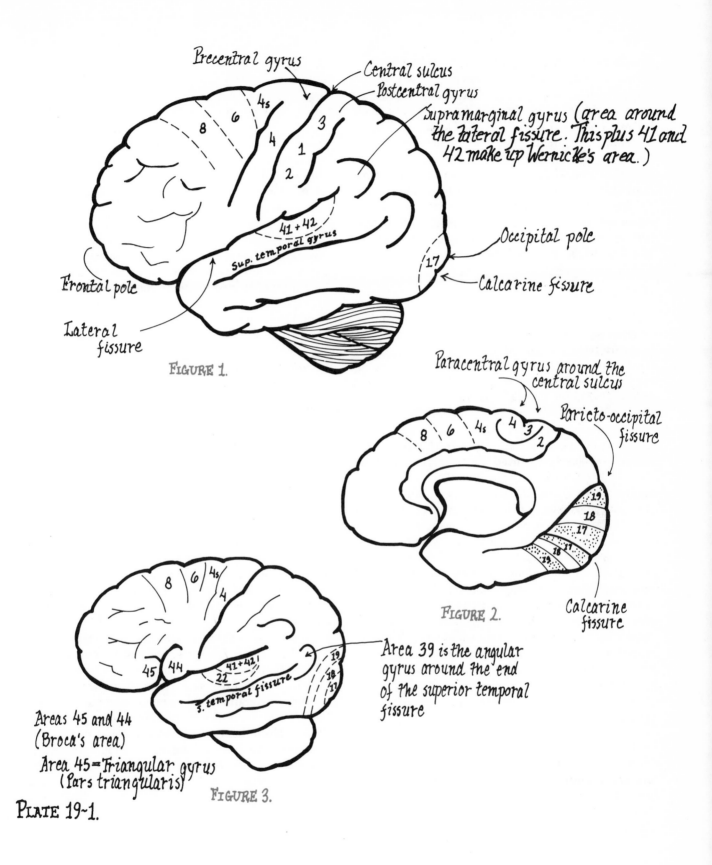

Precentral gyrus

Central sulcus

Postcentral gyrus

Supramarginal gyrus (area around
the lateral fissure. This plus 41 and
42 make up Wernicke's area.)

8   6   4s

4   3

1

2

41 + 42

Sup. temporal gyrus

Occipital pole

17

Calcarine fissure

Frontal pole

Lateral
fissure

FIGURE 1.

Paracentral gyrus around the
central sulcus

Parieto-occipital
fissure

8   6   4s   4   3
2

19
18
17
18
19

FIGURE 2.

Calcarine
fissure

8   6   4s
4

45   44   41 + 42
22
3. temporal fissure

19
18
17

Area 39 is the angular
gyrus around the end
of the superior temporal
fissure

Areas 45 and 44
(Broca's area)
Area 45 = Triangular gyrus
(Pars triangularis)   FIGURE 3.

PLATE 19~1.

69

the Greek word meaning "to know." Area 19 is concerned with automatic following movements of the eyes, which occur when an object, such as a jet, suddenly comes into the visual field and the eyes "lock in" and follow it. Associated with area 4 is area 4s, the suppressor band, and area 6, which helps with voluntary movements. Area 22 is the auditory association area. If this area is damaged on the dominant side (the left hemisphere is the dominant one for speech and language in most people, including those who are left-handed), the result is the condition known as *word deafness*, or *auditory aphasia*, which is discussed in the following section.

SENSORY (RECEPTOR) APHASIA

Aphasia is defined as the inability to understand or express the symbols connected with language; there are two basic kinds: sensory and motor. If one traces the superior temporal sulcus to its posterior end, the gray matter surrounding this end is the *angular gyrus* (area 39) of the parietal lobe (Figure 2). Damage to this area on the dominant cerebral hemisphere produces a condition known as *visual aphasia*, "word blindness," or *alexia*. In this condition the patient sees the printed words, but cannot read them—they are meaningless lines. This condition is equivalent to a Westerner looking at Chinese writing; all the Westerner sees are curved lines and characters that have no specific meaning.

Area 22, surrounding the primary auditory reception areas (41 and 42), is the auditory reception area. If it is damaged, again on the dominant cerebral hemisphere, *auditory aphasia* results. A patient with this condition experiences sound without any meaning—the same thing as when you hear speech in a completely foreign language. The patient can hear you speaking, but cannot understand what is being said. *Wernicke's aphasia* is a condition of both auditory and visual aphasia.

MOTOR APHASIA

On the inferior frontal gyrus, in the triangular and opercular regions, are found areas 44 and 45, also known as *Broca's area* (Figure 3). If these areas are injured in the dominant hemisphere in an adult,

they produce a condition in which the patient is unable to talk, even though the vocal muscles are not paralyzed. The patient knows what he or she wants to say, but all that comes out is garbled sound or one word repeated over and over again. One might speculate that the memory engrams connected with speech have been destroyed. If the damage occurs in childhood, the child can be taught to speak by utilizing the nondominant cerebral hemisphere.

APRAXIA

Apraxia is the inability to carry out purposeful, learned, voluntary acts although there is no paralysis present. It also involves the association areas. When told to take out his or her keys and open the door, the patient might pull out a coin or comb and try to put it into the keyhole. If the damage involves the loss of writing ability, it is known as *agraphia*.

AGNOSIA

Agnosia is the inability to recognize things even though one sees them. For example, a patient can walk down the street, see some broken glass in the way, and walk around it. However, when you ask what it is he walked around, the patient doesn't know.

These conditions may sound strange, but many things concerning the cerebral cortex are so. As can readily be appreciated, the subject of aphasias and apraxias, as well as other cerebral conditions such as epilepsy, are not as simple as has been presented here, but are very complex matters that have psychological aspects as well. Our "hard fact" knowledge is very restricted, and because experiments can't be performed easily on the human cortex, what little information we have comes from pathologic cases and autopsies. The reader who wishes to learn more about the telencephalon should consult *Correlative Anatomy of the Nervous System*, by Crosby, Humphrey, and Luer, which has nearly 200 pages on the subject and over 1,300 references. There are also books available that are devoted to individual subject matters, such as epilepsy and EEG.

Chapter 20

The Meninges

Brain tissue, having the consistency of a heavy pudding or custard, is the most delicate of all body tissues. For protection, this vital organ is located in a sealed bony chamber, the *skull*.* To protect it further from the rough bone and from blows and shocks to the head, the brain is enveloped by three membranes, called the *meninges*. The outermost covering is the tough, thick *dura mater*, which is adherent to the inner surface of the bone (Figure 1). In fact, it forms the periosteal layer of the calvarium. Beneath the dura mater is the middle covering, the thin and filamentous *arachnoid*. The third and innermost layer is the very thin, delicate, and capillary-rich *pia mater*, which is attached directly to the brain and dips down into the sulci and fissures (Figure 1).

Although the dura mater is closely applied to the inner bone surface, it can in certain instances separate from it, creating an area between the two known as the *epidural space* (see "Clinical Aspects" at the end of Chapter 21). Between the dura mater and the underlying arachnoid is a very narrow subdural space filled with a small amount of serous fluid that acts as a lubricant, preventing adhesion between the two membranes (Figure 1). Separating the arachnoid from the pia mater is a relatively large gap, the *subarachnoid space* that is filled with cerebrospinal fluid (CSF; Figure 1). This clear, lymph-like fluid fills the entire subarachnoid space and thus surrounds the brain with a protective cushion that absorbs shock waves to the head. As a further means of protection there are fibrous filaments known as the *arachnoid trabeculations*, which extend from the arachnoid to the pia and help "anchor" the brain to prevent it from excess movement in cases of sudden acceleration or deceleration (Figure 1). In the fluid-filled subarachnoid space are situated the cerebral arteries and veins (Figure 1). The pia mater is so closely attached to the underlying brain that there is no space, potential or otherwise, between the two. In this manner the pia mater acts as a restraining agent that holds the brain tissue together and prevents it from separating.

The dura mater dips down into the median longitudinal fissure, and this dural fold, lying between the cerebral hemispheres, is called the *falx cerebri* (Figures 1 and 2; see also Appendix III, Figures 2–5). The dura also dips into the space between the cerebellum and the overlying occipital lobes forming the *tentorium cerebelli* (Figures 1 and 2), a tent-like covering over the cerebellum. Finally, the dura mater dips between the two cerebellar hemispheres to form the *falx cerebelli* (Figure 2). All the meninges, the subarachnoid space, and the CSF pass through the foramen magnum at the base of the skull (Figure 1) and extend down the vertebral canal to enclose the spinal cord and nerves. In the vertebral canal the spinal cord most often ends at the level of the second or third lumbar vertebra. However its surrounding pia extends down as the filum terminale, which is attached to the coccygeal ligament that serves to anchor the spinal cord (Figure 3). In addition the pia mater has, on each side of the entire cord, tooth-like extensions called the dentate ligaments (Figure 3). These are attached to the arachna and dura and also serve to anchor and stabilize the spinal cord. All the spinal nerves, including those of the caudal equina, are covered by pia mater, and upon exiting they "pick up" the arachna and dura (Figure 3).

CLINICAL ASPECTS

Meningitis is an infection of the meninges; usually it is the arachnoid and pia mater that are attacked (leptomeningitis). As you probably know from personal experience, an infected and inflamed area is very sensitive, and any pressure or stretching of it causes great pain. In meningitis, when there is an attempt to flex (bend) the neck and thereby stretch the meninges, the muscles of the neck contract strongly to prevent the bending and subsequent pain. This phenomenon of muscle contraction to prevent stretching of inflamed structures is known as *guarding*. In cases of suspected meningitis, the physician tries to bend the neck of the supine patient. If the neck cannot be bent or if bending is accompanied by pain, this is a key sign that meningitis is probably present.

*The English word "skull" comes from the Scandinavian word "skulla" and the drinking toast sköl is also a derivative. The Vikings used to cut off the top part of their victims' skulls, invert them, and use them as drinking cups in their victory celebrations. The rounded top part of the skull is called the calvarium; the most famous derivative in history was located a short distance from the author's home in Jerusalem—Calvary, the rounded little hill on which Jesus was crucified.

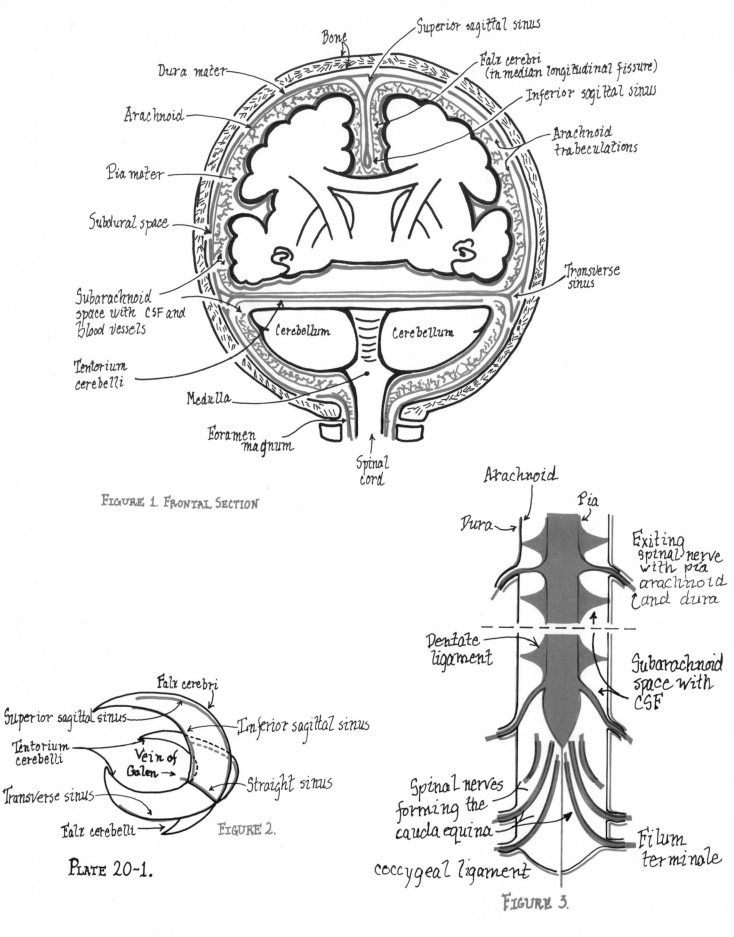

Bone

Superior sagittal sinus

Dura mater

Falx cerebri
(in median longitudinal fissure)

Inferior sagittal sinus

Arachnoid

Arachnoid
trabeculations

Pia mater

Subdural space

Transverse
sinus

Subarachnoid
space with CSF and
blood vessels

Cerebellum

Cerebellum

Tentorium
cerebelli

Medulla

Foramen
magnum

Spinal
cord

FIGURE 1. FRONTAL SECTION

Falx cerebri

Superior sagittal sinus

Inferior sagittal sinus

Tentorium
cerebelli

Vein of
Galen

Transverse sinus

Straight sinus

Falx cerebelli

FIGURE 2.

PLATE 20-1.

Dura

Arachnoid

Pia

Exiting
spinal nerve
with pia
arachnoid
and dura

Dentate
ligament

Subarachnoid
space with
CSF

Spinal nerves
forming the
cauda equina

coccygeal ligament

Filum
terminale

FIGURE 3.

Chapter 21

Blood Supply to the Brain

As mentioned in Chapter 1, nerve cells do not regenerate. They also need a constant, adequate supply of blood, and any interruption of it or injury to the vascular tree can quickly lead to irreparable lifelong damage or death. Because such injuries are commonly encountered in medical practice, knowledge and understanding of CNS vascularity are essential. Two pairs of arteries, the vertebrals and the internal carotids, are the only suppliers of blood to the brain. The *vertebral arteries* enter the skull through the foramen magnum and pass along the ventral surface of the medulla (Figure 1). After giving off the *anterior* and *posterior spinal arteries* as well as the *posterior inferior cerebellar artery*, they join together to form the *basilar artery*, which passes up to the beginning of the pons, where it bifurcates into the *posterior cerebral arteries*. These sweep back to supply the posterior part of the cerebral hemispheres, especially the medial and basilar surfaces (Figures 1, 2, and 3). In its course the basilar artery gives off the *anterior inferior cerebellar artery, pontine branches*, and the *superior cerebellar artery.*

The internal carotid arteries enter the skull through the foramen lacerum and lie adjacent to the lateral border of the optic chiasma (Figure 1). Here they bifurcate into the *anterior* and *middle cerebral arteries*. The anterior cerebral arteries pass forward into the medial longitudinal fissure and then sweep back to the parieto-occipital fissure, thus supplying the medial surface of the hemisphere (Figures 1–3). The *middle cerebral arteries* pass laterally between the temporal and frontal lobes. They emerge at the lateral fissure and fan out to supply most of the lateral surface of the hemisphere (Figures 1 and 2). In their course between the temporal and frontal lobes, the middle cerebral arteries give off the very important *striate arteries*, which help supply the internal capsule with its descending motor tracts (Figure 1). Because the striate arteries are the frequent site of cerebrovascular accidents (CVA), they are known as the "arteries of stroke."

The anterior cerebral arteries are connected to each other by the *anterior communicating artery.* There is also a posterior artery that links the middle cerebral artery with the posterior cerebral artery (Figure 1). Thus, at the base of the brain an anastomotic ring is formed between the vertebral and internal carotid arteries. This ring is called the *circle of Willis* and is important clinically because if one of the arteries becomes occluded, the blood can pass around to reach the deprived area, a phenomenon known as collateral circulation. In addition, the circle of Willis is a frequent site for *aneurysms.* An aneurysm forms when blood pressure at a weakening in the wall causes the artery to balloon out. This can press on adjacent structures, such as the optic chiasma, causing visual disturbances (Figure 1, and also refer to Chapter 15), or if it bursts can cause a CVA.

VENOUS DRAINAGE

Venous blood takes a roundabout circuit in its drainage to the neck. Most of the veins reach the surface of the brain and join larger veins. These cross the subarachnoid space and empty into large venous sinuses located within the dura mater. The superior cerebral veins drain into the superior sagittal sinus, whereas the inferior cerebral veins drain into the tranverse sinus, as well as the superficial middle cerebral vein (Figure 4). In addition there are anastamotic veins that connect the superficial middle cerebral vein with the sinuses (Figure 4). Blood from the center of the brain flows into the deep cerebral veins and then into the straight sinus. There is a confluence of these sinuses into each other: the superior sagittal and straight sinuses flow into the transverse, which continues into the sigmoid, which drains into the internal jugular vein of the neck. The superficial middle cerebral vein flows into the cavernous sinus located at the base of the brain (see Appendix III, Figure 5), and because of its location and the structures found in it (cranial nerves III, IV, V, VI), an infection of the cavernous sinus is very dangerous.

CLINICAL ASPECTS

If an artery becomes occluded by an embolism or through vasospasm, the area distal to the occlusion is deprived of its blood supply and the cells quickly die. This usually results in a stroke, the severity of which depends on the artery stopped and the site of occlusion, as well as other factors. Stroke can also occur if an artery ruptures, and, if the hemorrhage is massive, death can occur very quickly. After 3–4

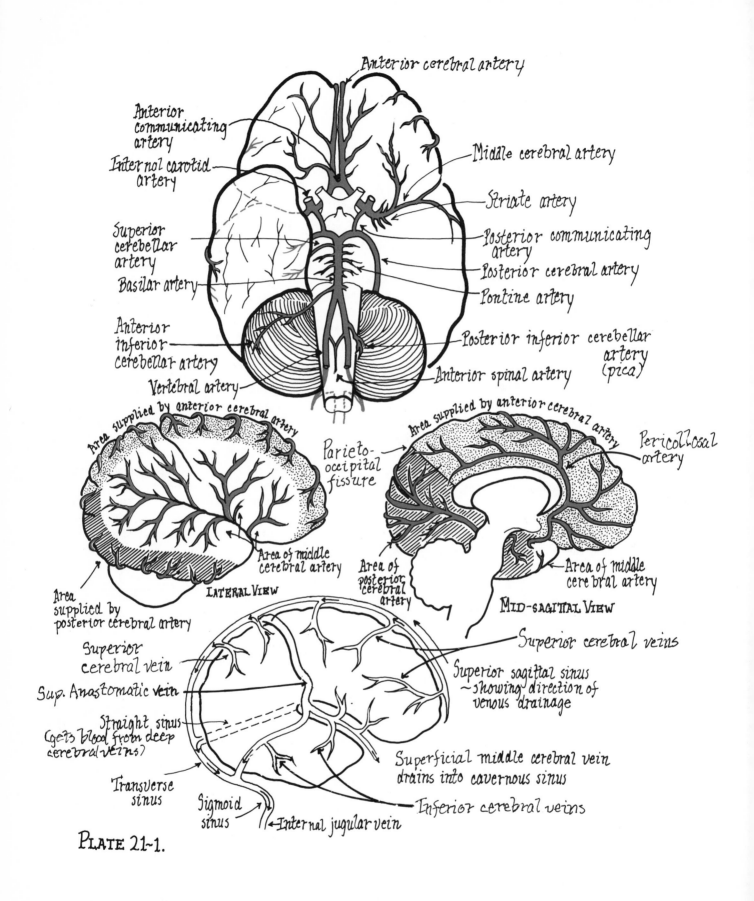

Anterior cerebral artery

Anterior communicating artery

Internal carotid artery

Superior cerebellar artery

Basilar artery

Anterior inferior cerebellar artery

Vertebral artery

Middle cerebral artery

Striate artery

Posterior communicating artery

Posterior cerebral artery

Pontine artery

Posterior inferior cerebellar artery (pica)

Anterior spinal artery

Area supplied by anterior cerebral artery

Parieto-occipital fissure

Area of middle cerebral artery

Area supplied by posterior cerebral artery

LATERAL VIEW

Area supplied by anterior cerebral artery

Pericallosal artery

Area of posterior cerebral artery

Area of middle cerebral artery

MID-SAGITTAL VIEW

Superior cerebral vein

Sup. Anastomatic vein

Straight sinus (gets blood from deep cerebral veins)

Transverse sinus

Sigmoid sinus

Internal jugular vein

Superior cerebral veins

Superior sagittal sinus ~ showing direction of venous drainage

Superficial middle cerebral vein drains into cavernous sinus

Inferior cerebral veins

PLATE 21-1.

74

minutes of arterial deprivation, neurons begin to die, with those of the cerebral cortex being most sensitive and those of the lower "vegetative" or brainstem centers being hardier. Thus there can be a short halt in the cerebral blood flow and following resumption the individual is a "vegetable" for life because the neurons of the higher centers, such as personality, memory etc., have died whereas the lower, life-sustaining ones are still viable. Another way of illustrating the importance of the blood supply is that although the brain is only 2% of total body weight it uses 15–20% of total cardiac output.

The middle meningeal artery does not supply the brain, but the dura of the middle cranial fossa. It lies between the dura mater and the skull, and in cases of trauma to the head, as in car accidents, jagged bone splinters, especially from the inner part of the bone, can cut the artery, although the patient for the first hour or two may have no complaints or visible injuries. Arterial blood, which is under high pressure, flows out rapidly between the dura and the bone, forming a rapidly expanding pool (an *epidural* or *extradural hematoma*) that presses on the underlying brainstem that contains the cardiac and respiratory centers, as well as being the site for consciousness. Unconsciousness and a progressively deepening coma ensue, and therefore immediate surgical intervention to clamp the artery and drain

the blood is necessary to prevent death. (Appendix III, Figure 11). This condition and others are beautifully illustrated by Dr. Netter in the world-famous Ciba collection of atlases.

Because the veins of elderly people are less resilient and more fragile than in younger individuals, a mild blow to the head can cause a cerebral vein (especially one of the superior cervical veins at its junction with the superior sagittal sinus) to rupture slightly. Because venous pressure is low, seepage is very slow, and the blood usually accumulates between the dura and the arachnoid, forming what is known as a *subdural hematoma*. Weeks later, after the blow has been forgotten, the slowly expanding hematoma presses on the brain, causing *various insidious and nonspecific symptoms*, such as dizziness, headaches, apathy, falling, confusion, and drowsiness. Indeed this constellation of complaints and symptoms in an elderly person should immediately alert the physician to the possibility of this condition. (In the past the mental complaints occasionally resulted in the patients being sent to a psychiatric hospital). Today in the great majority of cases, a CT scan can accurately and easily pinpoint the condition.

Subdural hematomas may also occur in newborns, as great pressure on the head during delivery may rupture a cerebral vein.

Chapter 22

Cerebrospinal Fluid and the Ventricular System

Cerebrospinal fluid (CSF) is a clear fluid filling the entire subarachnoid space. It acts as a protective "liquid cushion" around the brain and spinal cord by absorbing shock waves from blows and falls. In addition, it is a valuable diagnostic aid: by means of a relatively simple procedure known as a spinal tap, the physician can obtain a fresh sample of the fluid, quickly examine it, and get an accurate picture of what is taking place within the skull and brain.

Deep inside the brain is a series of interconnecting chambers—the ventricular system—and it is here that CSF is produced. In each cerebral hemisphere there is a large space, the *lateral ventricle* (see Appendix III, Figures 2–5), which is made up of an *anterior horn*, lying in the frontal lobe; the *body* or main part, lying in the frontal and parietal lobes; a *posterior horn*, in the occipital lobe; and an *inferior horn*, which sweeps down into the temporal lobe (Figures 1 and 2). In each lateral ventricle there is a delicate, lace-like structure, the *choroid plexus* (Figure 3; see also Appendix III, Figure 3), which is composed of pia mater enveloped by the thin membranous ependyma. Due to diffusion and active transport, the CSF passes from the capillary-rich choroid plexus into the ventricular space; it is therefore similar to lymph. The accumulating CSF fills the lateral ventricles and then flows out of them via the interventricular *foramen of Monro* and into the third ventricle (see Appendix III, Figures 3 and 4). This narrow, slit-like space lies in the midline between the walls of the right and left diencephalon (Figures 1 and 2; see also Plates IV and VII in Appendix II). The choroid plexus in the third ventricle also produces CSF, and all of the fluid flows into the narrow aqueduct of Sylvius, located in the midbrain (Figures 1 and 2; see also Plates IV, X, and XI in Appendix II). The aqueduct then empties into the fourth ventricle, in the pons and medulla (Figures 1, 2, and 3; see also Plate IV in Appendix II and Figure 4 in Appendix III). Here also is the choroid plexus, which produces CSF. In the thin roof of the fourth ventricle are three openings—the medial *foramen of Magendie* and the two lateral *foramina of Luschka*.* It is through these

openings that the CSF leaves the ventricular system and flows into and completely fills the subarachnoid space around the brain and cord (Figures 2 and 3). In certain regions the arachnoid is situated far from the pia mater, and the enlarged subarachnoid space forms areas known as *cisterns*; for example the cisterna magna (Figure 3 and Appendix IV, Figure 2).

An important question is: If CSF is constantly being produced, what happens to the excess fluid? In the area of the superior sagittal sinus, the arachnoid projects through small openings in the dura mater into the sinus. The accumulating CSF creates a pressure that forces the excess fluid out of the arachnoid projections and into the dural venous blood, which carries it away (Figures 3 and 4). In gross preparations these fine arachnoid projections resemble granules of sugar or salt and are therefore called *arachnoid granulations*.

CLINICAL ASPECTS

Hydrocephalus

Most often in newborn infants, a blockage may form somewhere in the ventricular system. Consequently, the CSF is unable to flow out and instead accumulates in the ventricles, where it presses on the nervous tissue, causing a thinning out of the brain with a widening of the ventricles (see Appendix III, Figure 8). Because the cranial bones of the baby have not yet fused, the expanding, fluid-filled brain separates the bones, and the head enlarges tremendously. The exact cause of hydrocephalus is unknown, but it may be due to failure of the foramina or aqueduct to develop, or they may become blocked by a tumor, following *encephalitis* (infection of the brain), or through inadequate CSF resorption into the venous sinuses. Therefore, examination of infants must include a measurement of the circumference of the head, and if it exceeds normal limits then diagnostic tests should be done.

Today excellent therapeutic results are obtained in the treatment of hydrocephalus by neurosurgically implanting a tube (catheter) from the anterior

---

*Magendie is *median*; Luschka is *lateral*.

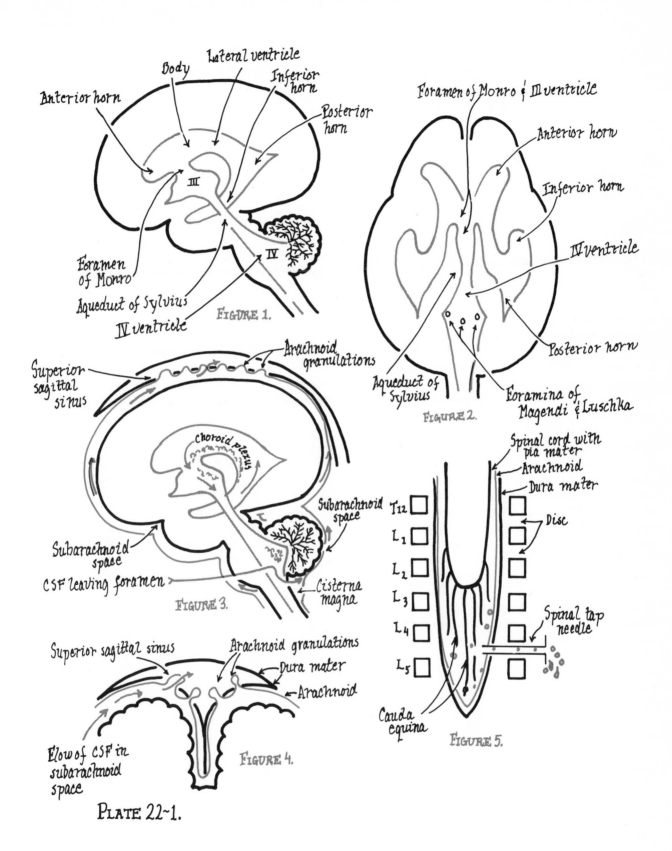

Anterior horn

Body

Lateral ventricle

Inferior horn

Posterior horn

Foramen of Monro

Aqueduct of Sylvius

IV ventricle

III

IV

FIGURE 1.

Foramen of Monro & III ventricle

Anterior horn

Inferior horn

IV ventricle

Posterior horn

Aqueduct of Sylvius

Foramina of Magendi & Luschka

FIGURE 2.

Superior sagittal sinus

Arachnoid granulations

choroid plexus

Subarachnoid space

Subarachnoid space

CSF leaving foramen

Cisterna magna

FIGURE 3.

Spinal cord with pia mater

Arachnoid

Dura mater

Disc

Spinal tap needle

T₁₂

L₁

L₂

L₃

L₄

L₅

Cauda equina

FIGURE 5.

Superior sagittal sinus

Arachnoid granulations

Dura mater

Arachnoid

Flow of CSF in subarachnoid space

FIGURE 4.

PLATE 22~1.

77

horn of the lateral ventricle to the abdominal (peritoneal) cavity. The excess CSF is thereby shunted off and absorbed in the pleural cavity.

Spinal Tap

Because the spinal cord is shorter than the vertebral column, it generally ends at the level of the first or second lumbar vertebra (Figure 5). Therefore, the subarachnoid space below this level can be tapped with no danger of injuring the cord. After giving a local anesthetic, the doctor inserts a sterile hollow needle in between the third and fourth or fourth and fifth lumbar vertebrae, punctures the dura mater, and enters the subarachnoid space filled with CSF. The hollow needle has a plunger, which is pulled out so that the CSF can then drip out. The physician first measures the pressure of the intracranial CSF, which normally can reach 200 mm of water. In certain brain diseases the CSF pressure is greatly elevated. However, one must *NEVER* attempt to reduce the pressure by letting out the CSF through a spinal tap, because the sudden downward flow of the released fluid pulls the brainstem into the foramen magnum, causing the almost instantaneous death of the patient.

The CSF obtained by spinal tap is examined grossly for pus or blood and microscopically for the presence of white blood cells, red blood cells, bacteria, and fungi. It is also examined for the levels of chloride, protein, and sugar. (In bacterial infections there is a decrease in sugar levels because it acts as a great energy source for the proliferating bacteria).

In certain operations in which general anesthesia is contraindicated, local anesthetic fluid can be injected through the spinal tap needle into the epidural or subarachnoid space, producing what is known as a sacral or lumbar block. The anesthetist employs techniques that prevent the anesthetic fluid from flowing up the vertebral canal and silencing nerves to vital organs.

Increased Intracranial Pressure

Many pathologic conditions (e.g., tumors, trauma, or CVAs) can produce an increase in intracranial pressure. This is often indicated by a patient's complaints of headaches, but it must be emphasized that most headaches are not the result of an increase in pressure. Increased intracranial pressure may be detected by looking with an ophthalmoscope into the patient's eye and observing the presence of papilledema of the optic disc of the retina. Normally, the optic disc is sharp and distinct, but when there is an increase in CSF pressure, papilledema results, (i.e., the borders of the disc become blurred, there is congestion or hemorrhage of the peripapillary veins, and the entire optic disc may bulge). The underlying cause should be sought and the pressure relieved in order to prevent brain damage, coma, or death.

After a spinal tap, some of the CSF may leak out into the surrounding tissues. This produces a decrease in intracranial pressure, which is often accompanied by headaches.

Chapter 23

Pathologic Conditions of the Central Nervous System

This chapter is designed to give the reader a short introductory overview of the most common neuro-pathologic conditions that he or she will encounter. In no way is it a substitute for a more detailed reading of the subject.

CEREBROVASCULAR ACCIDENT

Cerebrovascular accident (CVA) may be defined as damage to the brain as a result of a pathologic condition of the blood vessels, especially the arteries. CVAs, or strokes, are the third most common cause of death in the United States, after heart attacks and cancer, and nearly a million survivors are left disabled each year.

As mentioned in Chapter 1, the brain is very sensitive to oxygen deprivation. If the arterial supply to an area is cut off, it will undergo a process of degeneration and death, producing what is known as an infarcted area (see Appendix III, Figure 9). The arterial blockage may be the result of thrombus formation, emboli, or vasospasm and these cases account for 70–80% of all CVAs. The clinical picture that one sees depends on the area that is affected, but what is seen most often is some kind of upper motor neuron paralysis.

As one gets older the arteries become less elastic and more fragile; these changes, often combined with hypertension, can result in the rupture of a vessel. The subsequent *hemorrhage* (see Appendix III, Figure 10) often results in rapid death or permanent disablement.

An *aneurysm* is a local ballooning out of an arterial wall. Aneurysms in the brain are most often located in and around the circle of Willis and are known as berry aneurysms. Fifty percent arise from the internal carotid or middle meningeal arteries. Before rupture most berry aneurysms are asymptomatic, but if suspected they can be located and removed by microneurosurgery. If a berry aneurysm ruptures, there will be hemorrhaging into the subarachnoid space, followed often by rapid death. If the patient survives, he or she can be operated upon to remove the aneurysm.

TRANSIENT ISCHEMIC ATTACK

A transient ischemic attack (TIA) or "little stroke" in layperson's terms, occurs when a spasm or occlusion of a small artery causes an individual to lose consciousness briefly and then to recover with no paralysis. However the patient is confused and disoriented often has difficulty in speech and tongue movement. This condition can recur over a period of months or years.

INFECTIONS

Bacterial Infections

Meningitis is an infection of the cerebral and/or spinal meninges (usually the arachnoid and pia). In 80–90% of cases it is caused by one of three bacteria: *Neisseria meningitidis*, *Diplococcus pneumoniae*, or *Haemophilus influenzae* with the latter being the most frequent pathogen in children and infants. The triad of fever, headache, and stiff neck should immediately alert the physician to the possibility of the disease, and a spinal tap (lumbar puncture) should be done at once.

Brain abscess is a pocket or pockets of pus that have formed in the brain tissue (see Appendix III, Figure 12). They are rarely primary infections but mostly secondary ones from sites elsewhere in the body with the most common ones being middle ear infections, sinusitis, or purulent pulmonary conditions. The most common agents are *Staphylococcus*, *Streptococcus*, and *Pneumococcus*, and they spread by either direct extension or via the bloodstream. CT scanning has dramatically improved the correct diagnosis and treatment, which involves the use of antibiotics or surgical removal.

Tetanus occurs when a cut or wound is invaded by anaerobic *Clostridium tetani* or its spores. Once in the tissue, the bacteria produce a powerful neurotoxin that causes severe muscular spasms. The best "cure" is prevention by immunization.

Infection of the dural venous sinuses, like brain abscesses, is most often secondary to an infection elsewhere in the body. Because of its location at the base of the brain and the structures in it,* infection of the cavernous sinus is particularly dangerous.

Syphilis is caused by the spirochete *Treponema pallidum*. The last or tertiary stage of the illness occurs many years after the initial infection and may affect the nervous system, causing a multiplicity of symptoms, many of them mental (e.g., delusions of grandeur).

Botulism is a rare but headline-making form of food poisoning caused by the contamination of canned foods by the anaerobic bacteria, *Clostridium botulinus*. The exotoxin of this bacteria, one of the most powerful poisons known, attacks the neuromuscular junction, initially causing blurred or double vision and weakness of extraocular muscles. These symptoms are soon followed by dysarthria, dysphagia, and progressive weakening of musculature. Treatment is based on quick diagnosis and the use of antitoxins.

Viral Infections

Encephalitis is inflammation and infection of the brain tissue by any one of a large number of viruses. Among the most common types of encephalitis are St. Louis encephalitis, Eastern encephalitis, Japanese B encephalitis, and encephalitis lethargica. Mortality rates vary from type to type.

Poliomyelitis, once a highly prevalent and dreaded disease, specifically attacks the cell bodies of lower motor neurons, leaving in its wake a trail of death or paralysis. In the developed countries it has been eliminated by a vaccine developed by the great work of Enders, Salk, and Sabin.

Throughout history, *rabies* has been one of the most feared diseases, because once infected the patient always died, with death being preceded by the most terrifying symptoms, including excitability, refusal to drink water (hydrophobia) because of painful laryngeal spasms, and convulsions. The disease is transmitted via the saliva of a warm-blooded animal, such as a dog, cat, squirrel, or fox, that has been infected. The incubation period varies from 10 days to many months and sometimes more than a year. Animals that have bitten humans should be quarantined for 10 days. If the animal does not die during this period, it is not rabid. If the animal does die, the brain should be examined. Treatment consists of vaccination, but once symptoms have set in there is no cure or hope.

---

*Cranial nerves III, IV, V, VI and the internal carotid artery.

Fungus Infections

Fungal infections of the CNS are rare, but once established they are difficult to treat and the mortality rate is high. They often attack individuals whose immune system has been weakened or destroyed, (e.g., people taking immunosuppressive drugs, AIDS victims, etc.)

BRAIN TUMORS (NEOPLASMS)

Brain tumors may be derived from (1) nervous tissue, (2) nonnervous tissue of the CNS, or (3) from primary sites outside the CNS. Tumors of the last-named type are called metastatic in origin (see Appendix III, Figure 15). Malignancy does not depend only on the histology of the tumor cell but also on the location of the tumor. For example, a growth that is benign from a morphologic point of view may be so located that it cannot be reached surgically (e.g., a tumor in the midbrain) and will therefore be fatal.

Because neurons do not undergo mitosis, the vast majority of tumors derived from nervous tissue are glial in origin are known as *gliomas*. Gliomas constitute approximately 50–60% of all intracranial tumors. Histologically the most common are astrocytomas, which are graded on a scale of I–IV according to their malignancy. Type IV, the glioblastoma multiforme, is the most common and malignant type. Cerebral gliomas are rare in children, whereas cerebellar ones are the most common, often being situated in the roof of ventricle IV. Other gliomas include oligodendrocytomas, ependymomas, and the fast-growing medulloblastomas of the cerebellum that are found only in children, especially in the 4–8 age group. (Appendix III, Figure 16) About 30% of intracranial tumors arise from nonnervous tissue in the CNS, the most common being the slow-growing meningioma that is found most often in older people (Appendix III, Figure 13) Some other types of nonnervous intracranial tumors are the pinealoma; craniopharyngioma; accoustic schwannomas; angiomas; and pituitary adenomas (Appendix III, Figure 17).

Lastly tumors of the brain may be metastatic in origin (Appendix III, Figure 15), and these account for approximately 10% of all intracranial growths. In such cases, the main site of growth is in an organ, such as the lung or prostate, from which tumor cells have broken off and reached the brain via the circulatory system. To understand symptoms of tumors, it is helpful to remember:

1. Tumors are space-occupying lesions that also produce edema. Therefore they cause an increase in intracranial pressure that gives rise to *headaches*, *vomiting* (often projectile in nature), and/or *drowsiness*.
2. Tumors expand and *irritate* the brain matter, which in turn may cause *epileptic-like seizures*.
3. Tumors impinge on the brain and can therefore produce specific *(focal) signs* depending on where the tumor is located: if in the cerebellum, ataxia, falling, or other cerebellar signs may be caused; if in the frontal pole there may be personality changes or loss of smell (anosmia); and a pituitary adenoma can press on the optic chiasma and produce diplopia or other visual disturbances.

In the past the prognosis of brain tumors was poor, but with CT and MRI being able to reveal 95% of all intracranial growths, better surgical techniques, and chemotherapy the results now are much more favorable.

TRAUMA

In modern medical practice it is very common to see trauma to the brain and/or spinal cord from various causes, such as accidents (e.g., automobile, work, home, sports) and violence (e.g., blows, bullets, knife wounds). In these cases the skull and/or vertebral column is often fractured, and the delicate nervous tissue is compressed, lacerated, or destroyed, leading to death or permanent neurologic disabilities. Trauma to the brain is often accompanied by tearing of blood vessels, followed by hemorrhage and all the damage that it can produce.

Following an accident, clear or pink-tinged fluid seeping from the ear or nose often indicates a skull fracture with escaping CSF. A skull fracture may, however, exist without escaping CSF. Therefore, x-rays must be taken for confirmation.

DEMYELINATING DISEASES

In this group one finds multiple sclerosis (MS), which was discussed in Chapter 1. Also included is *postvaccinal encephalomyelitis*, which may occur, as its name indicates, after an individual has received a vaccination.

DEGENERATIVE DISEASES

Parkinsonism is a slow, progressive disease that affects older people, generally past the age of 50, and it has no known cause, cure, or means of prevention. Microscopically one sees a degeneration of the substantia nigra and the caudate or globus pallidus. The disease is characterized by resting tremors, marked hypertonicity of muscles that produce a mask-like face, and rigidity (see also Chapter 9).

Alzheimer's disease is the most common degenerative disease of older people. In recent years, it has assumed epidemic proportions, with an estimated 2½ million Americans affected by it; that figure is expected to rise. Microscopically one sees widespread neuronal death in the cerebral cortex. One also sees in the cortical neurons characteristic neurofibrillar masses and senile plaques. The cerebral hemisphere undergoes marked atrophy with a characteristic widening of the sulci and lateral ventricles that can be seen on a CT scan. The person afflicted with this disease forgets facts, speech, and the use of common everyday objects. Motor disabilities may cause the patient to become bedridden. On top of all this a slow progressive dementia generally appears with paranoia and hostility. Thus Alzheimer's disease, in addition to destroying the individual slowly, puts tremendous emotional, psychological, and financial strains on the family and society. Despite widespread research there is still no known cause, cure, or means of prevention for this disease.

TOXINS AND DRUGS

In this category are many exotic substances that are more often found in mystery and espionage stories than in real life, but when found in the latter they often outdo fiction.

Deaths from the venom of snakes, spiders, and scorpions are rare, but always stir the imagination. A few years ago in California, a man was convicted of attempted murder for placing a rattlesnake in the mailbox of his intended victim, who barely survived after reaching in to get the morning mail.* Some venoms are neurotoxins that depress the cardiac and/or respiratory centers, whereas others prevent the transmission of nervous impulses.

Heavy metals can also be lethal. Lead poisoning occurs most often in children, especially those in poor urban areas, who often chew on lead-based paint that has peeled from walls. Symptoms occur a few weeks after ingestion and are varied, insidi-

---

*The author disclaims responsibility for planting this idea, or any like it, in the minds of his readers.

ous, and nonspecific. They may include loss of appetite, irritability, loss of alertness, and, later, drowsiness, seizures, and coma. Mercury, manganese, and arsenic, as well as many industrial compounds, can cause neuropathy. For this reason, an accurate, detailed history of a patient's occupation, habitat, and other factors is very important. Finally, there are plant neurotoxins from curare, ergot, and some species of mushrooms.

Fifteen thousand people in the United States die every year from barbiturate poisoning—it is the leading cause of toxic death. By contrast, in 1979 there were only five reported cases of rabies, yet rabies is a far more terrifying word than barbiturates. Because barbiturate deaths are mostly self-inflicted, it would be far better if physicians would instead prescribe chloral hydrate, because it is one of the oldest, best, and safest hypnotics.

So much has already been written about heroin and cocaine that nothing can be added here that will enlighten or help the reader.

ALCOHOLISM

Alcoholism is one of the most prevalent diseases in the United States: an estimated 12–15 million people are alcoholics or have a drinking problem. Alcoholism has many causes and a strong genetic predisposition is involved.** Most of us have seen the havoc it wreaks upon the individual, the family, and society. There is no known cure, but complete abstinence and joining Alcoholics Anonymous give the best chance for avoidance of relapse.

EPILEPSY

This is a common neurologic condition that affects over 1 million people in the United States. Once—and perhaps even now—a sense of shame was attached to epilepsy, but it is a disease like any other and many famous people in history had a form of epilepsy, including Old Testament prophets, Julius Caesar, Dostoyevski, Byron, Alexander the Great, Peter the Great, and Pascal.

Epilepsy is characterized by sudden, uncoordinated discharges from cerebral neurons. The seizures have many forms and are categorized in vari-

ous ways, but about 95% of all seizures fall into two main groups: I, the general seizure and II, the partial seizure. In the first category are the grand mal and petit mal seizures. In the grand mal seizure the individual first has a visual or olfactory aura and loses consciousness. The entire body is then racked for 3–4 minutes by severe, tonic-clonic muscular contractions; foaming of saliva at the mouth; and interruption of breathing with cyanosis—a truly frightening sight to the unexperienced.

Petit mal epilepsy occurs most often in children between the age of 4 and puberty. The seizures consist of a loss of consciousness lasting from 1–3 seconds without closure of the eyes or any muscle spasms. In fact, the child is often unaware of his or her condition, and the child's teachers may complain that the pupil often doesn't pay attention and is daydreaming. An EEG is very useful in reaching a diagnosis. In most cases the symptoms disappear after puberty but if they do not, the petit mal seizure frequently evolves into the grand mal type.

The partial seizures often have a physical cause, such as a glial scar or tumor that acts as a cerebral irritant and center for electrical discharge. There are also two main types of partial seizures—the psychomotor and the focal. In the psychomotor, which is sometimes called temporal lobe epilepsy, the patient first has visual or olfactory hallucinations followed by altered states of consciousness, but does not lose consciousness. These altered states of consciousness involve such psychic phenomena as feelings of unreality or déja vu (familiarity) combined with anxiety. The attack then usually ends with some inappropriate motor phenomena.

The focal or Jackson seizure starts from a generally known motor focus on the precentral gyrus, and one sees such manifestations as finger jerks, and dorsiflexion of the foot.

Lastly, high fever in some infants and children produces seizures.

Although much research has been and is being done, the cause of epilepsy is still unknown in most cases. However, in some cases, there is a definite physical focus, such as a glial scar or tumor. Fortunately, in the majority of cases epileptic seizures can be prevented completely by the use of proper anticonvulsive drugs.

METABOLIC DISEASES

Metabolic diseases of the CNS are divided into two main groups: the acquired and the inherited. The

---

**An interesting research paper on this topic is: Goodwin, D., et al. Alcohol problems in adoptees raised apart from alcoholic parents. Archives of General Psychiatry 28:238, 1973.

former are really metabolic diseases of other organs that secondarily affect the brain. For example, hypothyroidism in children (cretinism) produces, among other things, severe mental retardation. Hypoglycemia can also adversely affect the brain. Recently in New York City a man was convicted of having attempted to murder his wealthy socialite wife by injecting her with a massive dose of insulin. She survived, but is in a coma and doctors fear she will remain so for the rest of her life. In a retrial the husband was acquitted of the charges. Because the liver is a vital organ involved in the metabolic process, damage to it can produce CNS symptoms that may end in coma and death.

The inherited or inborn metabolic diseases are due to an enzyme defect that produces an abnormal metabolism of various substances. As there are now over 100 such diseases, many with such quaint names as gargoylism and maple syrup urine disease, only the most common are mentioned here.

In *phenylketonuria* (PKU) there is an absence of the enzyme phenylalanine hydralase, which normally converts phenylalanine to tyrosine. In its absence, and if not detected and treated in time, the phenylalanine accumulates in the body and will produce neurologic and mental symptoms. Characteristic laboratory findings include phenylpyruvic acid present in the urine and elevated levels of serum phenylalanine.

Tay-Sachs disease is an autosomal recessive disease seen almost exclusively (95%) in Jewish children with an Eastern European background. Due to an absence of hexosaminidase A, there is an accumulation of lipids known as gangliosides in the brain cells. The disease begins in infancy and, there being no known means of prevention or cure, ends fatally by age 3 or 4. A cherry-red macula is a pathognomonic sign of this illness.

Infantile Goucher's disease manifests itself in the first half-year of life. Due to faulty fat metabolism, there is a buildup of cerebrosides in the cells of bone marrow, liver, and spleen, as well as in the brain. Large histiocytes known as Goucher cells are characteristic microscopic findings in this condition. There is no known cure, and the disease runs a progressively downhill course.

CONGENITAL DEFECTS

Congenital neuropathologic conditions may arise from a number of different causes, including genetic disorder, radiation, anoxia, and maternal in-

fections. *Down's syndrome (mongoloidism)* is due to genetic disorder in the child, and there is a much higher incidence of it in women over 40 who become pregnant.

A pregnant woman may get a rubella infection, which is a very mild thing for her. However, the virus may also attack the fetus, causing the child to be born deaf. In a pregnant woman who is also a drug addict, the heroin passes the placental barrier, and the unborn child may become addicted. After birth, the child is cut off from the source of the drug, and severe withdrawal signs are seen. Also, in the pregnant woman who smokes, the nicotine and other byproducts pass the placental barrier to affect the fetus adversely.

Finally there are many neurologically relevant conditions that have no known cause. Among them are dyslexia, stammering, spina bifida, mental retardation, and anencephaly (failure of the forebrain or brain to develop). *Dyslexia* (word blindness) is the inability or difficulty in recognizing letters, reading words, spelling, or writing, although the individual is neurologically healthy and is often very bright and intelligent. The condition tends to run in families with four to five times as many males affected as females. It is now realized that undetected dyslexia may be one reason a student does poorly in school. Also very poor writing, avoidance of reading, and reading upside down or sideways may indicate the presence of dyslexia. Once detected, intensive private tutoring helps improve the student's performance.

Stammering is a world-wide, ancient* condition that once again affects males more than females by a ratio of 4:1. Many children have periods in their life when they stammer, but the majority outgrow it. There are numerous theories of causation and many forms of therapy, but their results are very poor and disappointing. Stress generally worsens the condition, but most if not all stammerers are fluent in some situations, such as when they are singing. One of the best actors the author ever saw stammered in private life, but on stage was perfectly articulate and gave superb performances.

Spina bifida is a congenital malformation that occurs in about 1/1000 births in which the arches of one or several vertebra, usually in the lumbosacral

---

*Moses (see Exodus 4: 10–16), the Roman Emperor Claudius and King George VI of England, Prince Charles' grandfather, all were stammerers.

region, have failed to develop or fuse in the midline. In some cases there is no protrusion of the meninges, but in others they protrude and push up under the skin, often forming a rounded sac known as a *meningocele* (Appendix III, Figure 18). If in addition to the meninges, the cord and/or the spinal nerves also push out, the result is then called a *meningomydocele*.

MYASTHENIA GRAVIS

This is an insidious disease characterized by intermittent weakness of voluntary muscle, especially the muscles of the eyelid, face, jaw, and limbs. As a result the patient has ptosis, drooping jaw, difficulties in swallowing and speech, and changes in facial expression. It was mentioned in Chapter 1 that the junction between the axon and the voluntary muscle is the motor end plate and that the neurotransmitter is acetylcholine. This reacts with the acetylcholine receptor site to cause transmission of nerve impulses and contraction. Then an enzyme, acetylcholine esterase, breaks down acetylcholine, enabling the motor end plate and muscle fiber to repolarize and be ready to contract again. If repolarization didn't occur then the contracted muscle would eventually become fatigued and paralysis would follow.

Recent research has shown that myasthenia gravis is an auto-immune disease. The acetylcholine receptor sites on the motor end plate are proteins, and in some individuals they act as antigens, producing antibodies that react with and destroy many of the receptor sites and reduce the efficiency of many others. The amount of acetylcholine released is normal, but because the number and efficiency of sites are lowered, muscles are weakened and they tire quickly. Treatment consists of prolonging the life of acetylcholine by giving neuromuscular blocking agents, such as physostigmine or edrophonium, which block the acetylcholine esterase that breaks down acetylcholine.

Clinically there are three kinds of neuromuscular blocking agents, and each has its own characteristics and medical application. The first kind is exemplified by curare, a drug used by South American Indians (and mystery writers) to kill their prey and enemies. It is a powerful poison that blocks neuromuscular transmission by competitive inhibition; that is, the curare molecules, rather than acetylcholine, occupy the receptor sites on the motor end

plate. Paralysis of voluntary muscles, including those of respiration, occurs and is quickly followed by death. In general surgery, muscles, especially those of the abdomen, must be relaxed for the surgeons to operate but they are often tense and hard and you'll hear the surgeon say to the anesthetist that the patient "is too tight." The latter then gives small measured doses of curare to relax the muscles but not enough to cause paralysis.

Succinylcholine, an example of the second kind of blocking agent causes prolonged depolarization of the motor end plate, and one therefore sees initial muscle contraction followed by flaccid paralysis. Clinically it is used in general surgery to relax muscles. It is also virtually undetectable, being the closest thing to a perfect poison and, not surprisingly, was at the center of one of the most sensational murder cases in the United States in the 20th century. Dr. Coppolino, an anesthetist, was tried and found guilty of murdering his wife by injecting her with a large dose of succinylcholine in order to marry his mistress. (Six months before this case, he was tried but acquitted on the charge of murdering by suffocation the husband of yet another mistress. In this first case, everything hung on the condition of the cricoid cartilage in the neck—was it broken before or after the murder?) For fascinating accounts of these trials, one from the prosecution's point of view and the other through the eyes of the defense, I suggest you read: *Autopsy—the Memoirs of the World's Greatest Medical Detective* by Milton Halpern, M.D. who was the major prosecution witness in both cases and *The Defense Never Rests* by F. Lee Bailey who defended Dr. Coppolino in both his trials. In addition to these cases both books have other interesting cases in which medical evidence was the crucial factor—in short, real-life "Quincy" at its best. (Both books are published by Signet Pocket Books.)

The third and last type of neuromuscular blocking agent works by "knocking out" or neutralizing acetylcholine esterase, thereby producing a buildup of acetylcholine. The best example of these antiacetylcholine esterases are neostigmine and physostigmine, which are used in the treatment of myasthenia gravis and which are classified as reversible agents. In addition there are certain organophosphorus anticholinesterases whose action is irreversible and which are used to make the deadly nerve gases. These cause the muscles to contract (muscle fasciculation) initially; muscle paralysis and death then follow. The main antidote to these gases is the quick injection of atropine.

TEENAGE SUICIDE

In the last few years the teenage suicide rate in the United States has risen sharply to a point where it is one of the greatest causes of death in this age group—about 5000 fatalities each year. Although there are psychological factors at work one must also keep in mind the biological ones: that this is the period in life of the greatest turmoil and stress; that these have an organic basis, i.e. the hormonal secretions which cause a surge in sexual and aggressive feelings. Also there are known substances whose ingestion can cause depression followed by suicide,* and we still know very little about the body chemistry of depression. Finally, there is the known fact that the majority of teenage suicides are white males. Research is now being done to better clarify the nonpsychological (organic) factors of depression and how they interact with the psychological ones. It would be wise to keep in mind Freud's dictum: "we must recollect that all our provisional ideas in psychology will someday be based on an organic substructure" (from Chapter III of "On Narcissism"). The successful use of lithium in the treatment of manic-depressive psychosis gives much support to his statement.

---

*In the late 1940s U.S. scientists working for certain government agencies administered to some individuals, without their consent or awareness, some of these substances. The individuals so dosed went into deep depressions and committed suicide within 24 hours. The government admitted its errors and paid compensation to the families of the victims.

Special Neuroanatomic and Neuropharmacologic Glossary

WORD	DERIVATION	ILLUSTRATIVE EXAMPLE OR COGNATE
Agnosia	*a*, not *gnosis*, knowledge	Agnostic
Alexia	*a*, not *lexis*, word	Lexicon
Algia-	pain	Analgesic; nostalgia, the mental pain of returning or going back.
Aqueduct	*aqua*, water *ductus*, a leading	Aquarium; duke, "a leader"
Archi-	ancient	Archeology
Arachnoid	*arachne*, spider *eidos*, resemblance	The arachnoid resembles a cobweb.
Arcuate	*arcus*, a bow	Arch; archery
Astrocyte	*astron*, star kytos, cell	Astronomy
Ataxia	*a*, not *taxia*, orderly	Taxonomy
Ballism	to throw	Ball, ballistics
Brachium	*brachium*, arm	Embrace
Carotid	*karoo*, to put to sleep	Pressure on the carotid artery results in unconsciousness, as is well known in judo.
Caudate	*cauda*, a tail	A caudate nucleus has a tail.
Cerebellum	*Cerebellum* is the diminutive of *cerebrum* (brain), and it means "little brain."	
Cerebrum	*cerebrum*, brain	Cerebration is thinking.
Chiasma	The Greek letter chi (χ) is cross-shaped.	A chiasma is an arrangement in the form of a crossing.
Chorea	*choreia*, dance	People afflicted with Huntington's chorea exhibit characteristic ("dancing") movements. Choreography
Cingulum	belt	Shingles (the disease) is a verbal corruption because the Herpes Simplex virus follows the path of the intercostal nerves and forms a belt-like welt of vescicles around the chest wall.
Cistern	*cisterna*, a well	
Claustrum	*claustrum*, enclosure	Claustrophobia; closet
Clinoid	bed post; the four clinoid processes were thought to resemble the four posts of a bed	Clinic
Cornu	horn	Cornucopia
Coronary	*corona*, crown or garland Also, the *corona radiata* is a fan shaped ("radiating") fiber mass in the cerebral cortex.	The coronary arteries encircle the heart. Coronation
Corpus callosum	*corpus*, body *callosum*, hard	Callus; corporation
Cortex	*cortex*, bark	The cerebral cortex covers the cerebral hemisphere, much as bark covers the trunk of a tree.
Crista	crest	
Cuneate	*cuneatus*, wedge-shaped	The cuneiform writing of ancient Babylon had wedge-shaped characters.
Decussation	The Roman numeral X is called *deca*.	A decussation is a crossing.

WORD	DERIVATION	ILLUSTRATIVE EXAMPLE OR COGNATE
Dendrite	*dendron*, branching figure or tree	Rhododendron
Dentate	*dens*, tooth *dentatus*, tooth-shaped	Dentist
Dura mater	*dura*, hard *mater*, mother	Durable; alma mater
Dyskinesia	*dis*, improper *kinesia*, motion	Disorder; disease; kinetics
Edema	swollen	Oedipus (see Appendix VI, "Did You Know"?)
Epi-	Greek prefix meaning "upon, over, above"	An epitaph is inscribed over a grave *(taphos)*.
Fasciculus	*fasciculus*, a bundle (of rods or fibers)	The symbol of the Italian Fascists was the Roman bundles of rods, the *fascis* seen on old Mercury head dimes.
Fornix	*fornix*, arch	In ancient Rome the prostitutes hung around the supporting arches of the viaducts. A man visiting the area was engaged in fornication.
Genu	*genu*, knee	Genuflect, i.e., bend (bow) before royalty
Glia	*glia*, glue	Glial cells "hold together" the neurons.
Glossal	*glossa*, tongue	Glossary
Gracilis	*gracilis*, slender	
Gyrus	*gyros*, ring, circle	Gyrate; gyroscope
Hippocampus	*hippus*, horse *campus*, sea	In cross-section this hippocampus resembles a sea-horse. Hippodrome
Hypo-	Greek prefix meaning "under, below"	A hypodermic goes under the skin *(dermis)*.
Insula	*insula*, island	Insulin is produced by the islands of Langerhans; insulation
Internuncial	*inter*, between *nuncio*, messenger	Announce; papal nuncio
Lamina	layer or thin plate	Lamination
Lemniscus	*lemniscus*, ribbon, band	*Lens* is the Latin word for lentil, the "lens-shaped" vegetable of the bean family.
Limbic	*limbus*, border or edge	Limbo is the area bordering on Hell.
Lingula	*lingula*, little tongue	Linguist; language
Lumbar	*lumbus*, loin or flank	Lumbago
Macula	spot	Immaculate, spotless, clean
Mamillary	*mamma*, breast	Mammary; mammals
Mesencephalon	*meso*, middle *encephalos*, the brain	Mezzanine
Oligodendroglia	*oligo*, few *dendron*, branching figure or tree *glia*, glue	Oligarchy, "a few who rule"
Paleo	old	Paleontology
Pallidus	*pallidus*, pale	The pallidus is pale in comparison to the neighboring putamen.
Peduncle	*ped*, foot, limb, stalk	Pedal; pedestrian
Petrous	rock	Petrified; refers to the "rock" on which the Catholic Church stands. Peter is also slang for penis.
Pia mater	*pia*, soft, delicate *mater*, mother	Pianissimo is a musical term meaning "very soft."
Pineal	*pinea*, pine cone	The pineal body is conical.
Pons	*pons*, bridge	Pontoon
Ramus	*ramus*, branch	Ramifications
Rectus	*rectus*, straight	Rectify; erect
Reticular	*reticulum*, small net	A reticle is the network of lines in a telescopic sight; a lady's reticule is a small net bag.
Rhinencephalon	*rhin*, nose *encephalos*, the brain	Rhinoceros
Rubro	*ruber*, red	Ruby
Sacral	*sacer*, holy, sacred	The sacral bone was believed to resist decomposition and thus serve as the basis for resurrection.

WORD	DERIVATION	ILLUSTRATIVE EXAMPLE OR COGNATE
Sagittal	*sagitta*, arrow	Sagittarius is the Archer of the zodiac.
Sella turcica	*sella*, saddle	The sella turcica resembles a Turkish saddle.
	turcica, Turkish	
Septum	*septum*, a partition	Separate
Substantia nigra	*substantia*, substance	Nigeria; negroid
	nigra, black	
Tapetum	*tapete*, carpet	Tapestry
Tectum	*tectum*, roof	Architecture
Temporal	*tempus*, time	The temporal area gives evidence of the passage of time; i.e., the hair turns gray.
Tentorium	*tentorium*, tent	
Tubercle	*tuber*, a swelling or rounded projection	Tubers (potatoes); protuberance
Vagus	*vagus*, wandering	The vagus nerve extends into the thorax and abdomen. Vagabond; vagrant
Velum	*velum*, covering	Veil
Venereal	*Venus*, the goddess of love	
Ventricle	*ventrus*, chamber, cavity, hollow, stomach	A ventriloquist "speaks from the stomach."
Vermis	*vermis*, worm	The cerebellar vermis resembles a worm. Vermin
Vertebra	*vert*, to turn	Vertigo; vertebra (they turn on themselves)

TERMS RELATED TO NEUROPHARMACOLOGY

Barbiturate	Emil Fisher first produced barbiturates by condensing malonic acid with urea. The correct name should be malonylurate. The urea was extracted from large quantities of urine given to him by a waitress who worked in a coffeehouse he frequented (coffee is a diuretic agent). Not surprisingly, her name was Barbara, and to thank her for her efforts on behalf of science, he named the new drug after her.
Belladonna	*Bella donna* is Italian for "beautiful lady." In Italy during the Renaissance, ladies before going to parties would put belladonna (atropine) in their eyes, causing the pupils to dilate and the eyes to sparkle, thus enhancing their beauty. However, the drug greatly blurred their vision, and one can imagine the scene that ensued when such a lady mistook her husband for her lover.
Cocaine	Cocaine comes from the leaves of the coca tree. Sigmund Freud discovered its use as a local anesthetic for the eye. For a while, he also used it to get "high," or "euphoric," as he put it.
Hashish	This is an Arabic word. In the Middle East during the Crusades, professional killers often smoked hashish before doing a "hit," and for this reason they were called *hash-ha-shans*. The Crusaders could not pronounce this guttural word and corrupted it to "assassins," from which we get the word "assassinate."
Heroin	This drug gets its name from the fact that it often gives one transitory heroic feelings.
Marijuana	This drug is so called from the belief that it is an aphrodisiac. It is derived from the Spanish names Maria, which is feminine, and Juan, which is masculine.
Morphine	Morpheus was the Greek god of dreams, and taking morphine puts one in a dream-like state. Shapes and forms appear in dreams, and from this is also derived the word morphology, meaning the study of structures or forms.
Nicotine	This drug was named after Jean Nicot, who introduced tobacco into France.

Appendix II

Atlas of the Brain

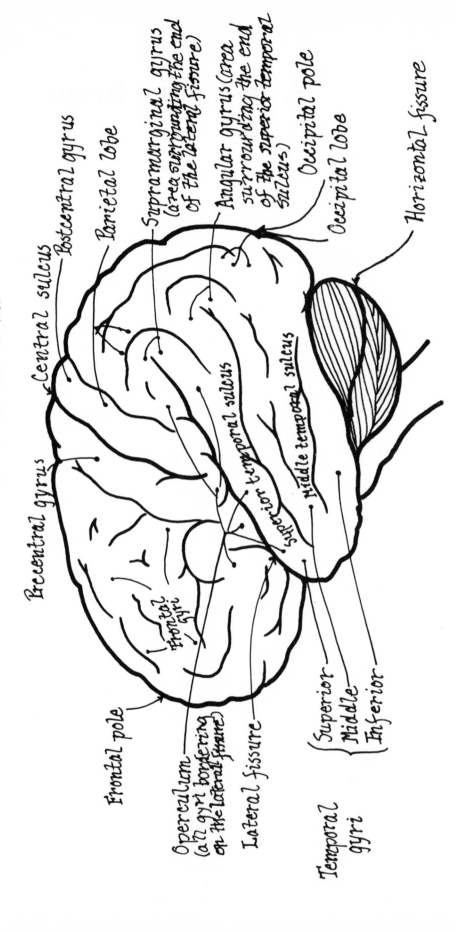

ATLAS PLATE I LATERAL VIEW OF THE BRAIN.

Precentral gyrus

Central sulcus

Postcentral gyrus

Parietal lobe

Supramarginal gyrus (area surrounding the end of the lateral fissure)

Angular gyrus (area surrounding the end of the superior temporal sulcus)

Occipital pole

Occipital lobe

Horizontal fissure

Frontal pole

Frontal gyri

Operculum (all gyri bordering on the lateral fissure)

Lateral fissure

Superior temporal sulcus

Middle temporal sulcus

Temporal gyri
{ Superior
  Middle
  Inferior }

ATLAS PLATE II BASAL VIEW OF THE BRAIN.*

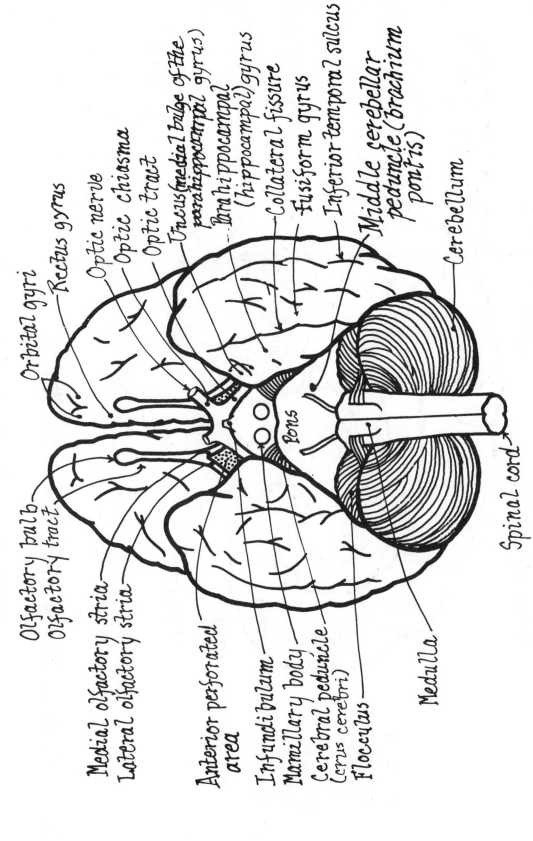

Olfactory bulb
Olfactory tract
Orbital gyri
Rectus gyrus
Optic nerve
Optic chiasma
Optic tract
Uncus(medial bulge of the parahippocampal gyrus)
Parahippocampal (hippocampal) gyrus
Collateral fissure
Fusiform gyrus
Inferior temporal sulcus
Middle cerebellar peduncle (brachium pontis)
Cerebellum

Medial olfactory stria
Lateral olfactory stria
Anterior perforated area
Infundibulum
Mamillary body
Cerebral peduncle (crus cerebri)
Flocculus
Medulla
Spinal cord

Pons

* For a more detailed view of the brainstem with the cranial nerves, see PLATE VII of this atlas.

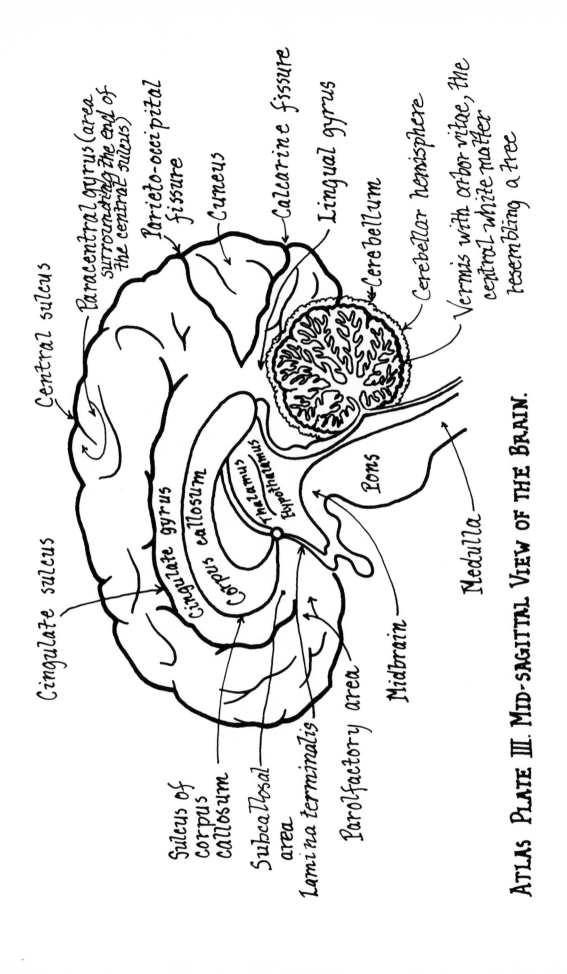

Central sulcus

Paracentral gyrus (area surrounding the end of the central sulcus)

Parieto-occipital fissure

Cuneus

Calcarine fissure

Lingual gyrus

Cerebellum

Cerebellar hemisphere

Vermis with arbor-vitae, the central white matter resembling a tree

Cingulate sulcus

Cingulate gyrus

Corpus callosum

Thalamus

Hypothalamus

Pons

Medulla

Midbrain

Parolfactory area

Lamina terminalis

Subcallosal area

Sulcus of corpus callosum

ATLAS PLATE III. MID-SAGITTAL VIEW OF THE BRAIN.

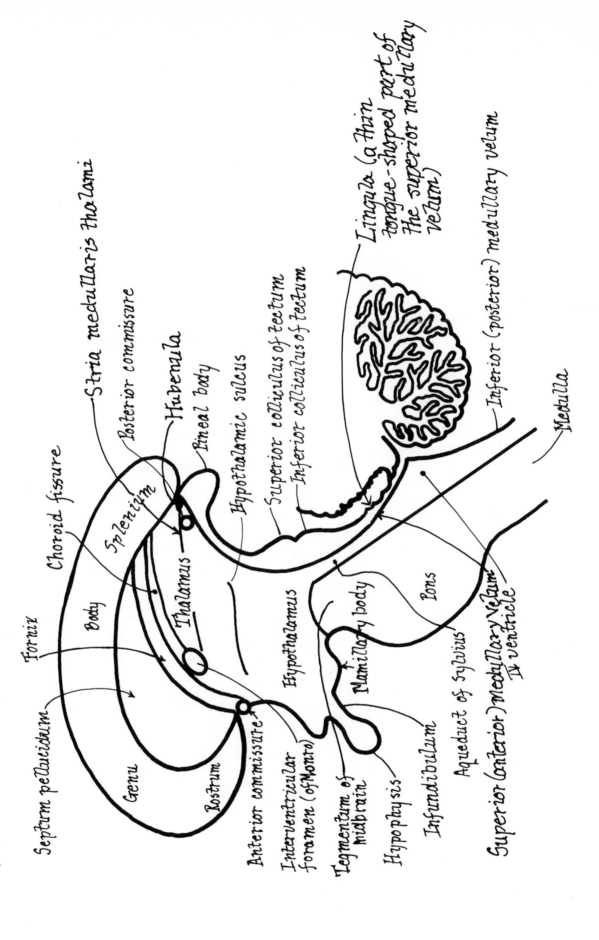

ATLAS PLATE IV. ENLARGED MID-SAGITTAL VIEW OF THE BRAIN.

Septum pellucidum

Fornix

Choroid fissure

Body

Genu

Rostrum

Stria medullaris thalami

Posterior commissure

Splenium

Habenula

Pineal body

Thalamus

Hypothalamic sulcus

Superior colliculus of tectum

Inferior colliculus of tectum

Lingula (a thin tongue-shaped part of the superior medullary velum)

Inferior (posterior) medullary velum

Medulla

Anterior commissure

Interventricular foramen (of Monro)

Hypothalamus

Tegmentum of midbrain

Mamillary body

Pons

Hypophysis

Infundibulum

Aqueduct of Sylvius

Superior (anterior) medullary velum
IV ventricle

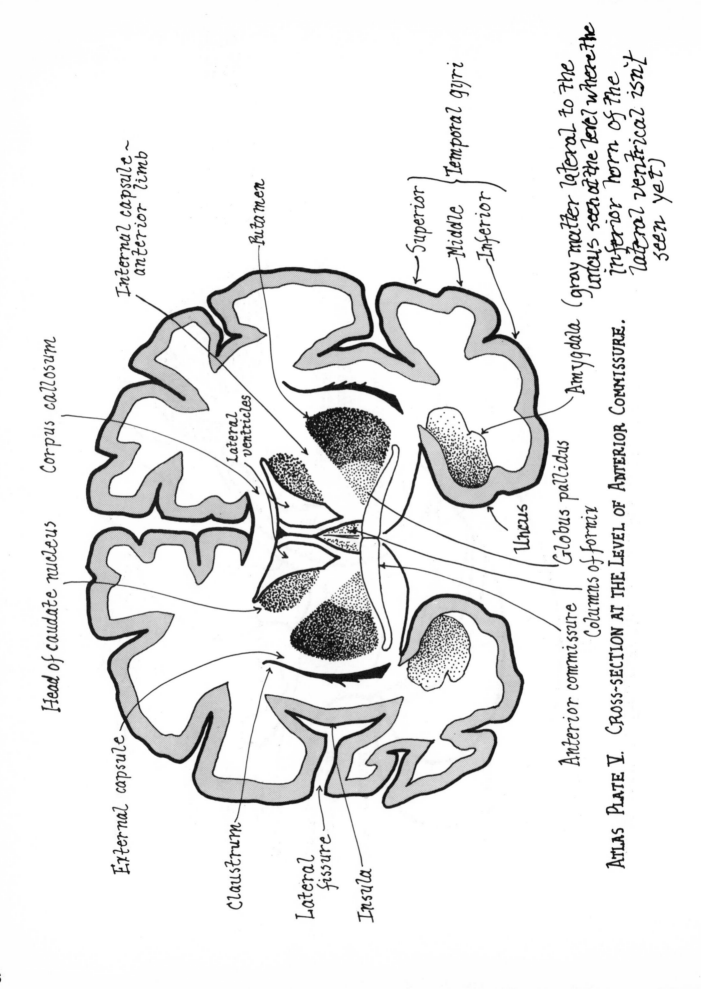

Head of caudate nucleus

Corpus callosum

Internal capsule ~ anterior limb

Putamen

Superior ⟍
Middle } Temporal gyri
Inferior ⟋

Lateral ventricles

Amygdala (gray matter lateral to the uncus; seen at the level where the inferior horn of the lateral ventrical isn't seen yet)

External capsule

Claustrum

Lateral fissure

Insula

Anterior commissure
Columns of fornix

Uncus

Globus pallidus

ATLAS PLATE V. CROSS-SECTION AT THE LEVEL OF ANTERIOR COMMISSURE.

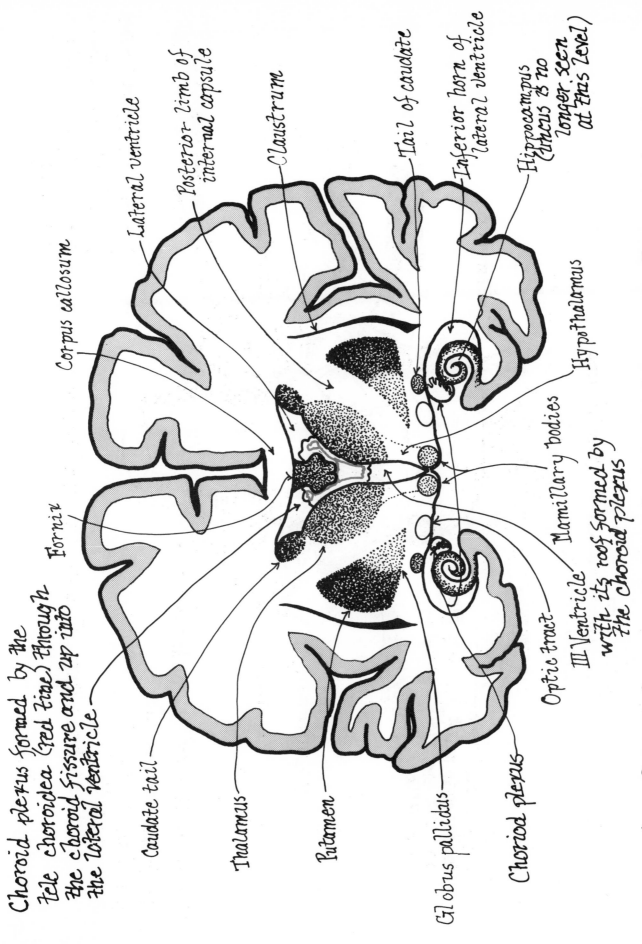

Choroid plexus formed by the
tele choroidea (red line) through
the choroid fissure and up into
the lateral ventricle.

Corpus callosum

Fornix

Caudate tail

Thalamus

Putamen

Globus pallidus

Choroid plexus

Optic tract

III Ventricle
with its roof formed by
the choroid plexus

Mamillary bodies

Hypothalamus

Lateral ventricle

Posterior limb of
internal capsule

Claustrum

Tail of caudate

Inferior horn of
lateral ventricle

Hippocampus
(uncus is no
longer seen
at this level)

ATLAS PLATE VI. CROSS-SECTION OF THE BRAIN AT THE LEVEL OF THE MAMILLARY BODIES.

97

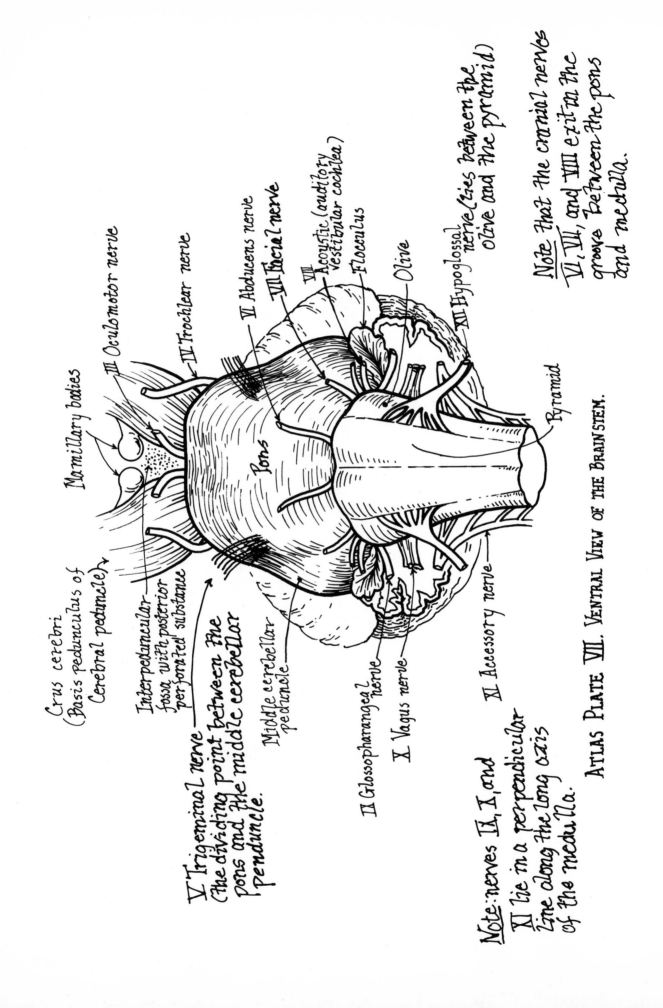

Crus cerebri
(Basis pedunculus of
Cerebral peduncle)

Mamillary bodies

Interpeduncular
fossa with posterior
perforated substance

V Trigeminal nerve
(The dividing point between the
pons and the middle cerebellar
peduncle.

Middle cerebellar
peduncle

IX Glossopharyngeal
nerve

X Vagus nerve

Note: nerves IX, X, and
XI lie in a perpendicular
line along the long axis
of the medulla.

XI Accessory nerve

III Oculomotor nerve

IV Trochlear nerve

VI Abducens nerve

VII Facial nerve

VIII

Acoustic (auditory
vestibular cochlea)

Flocculus

Olive

XII Hypoglossal
nerve (lies between the
olive and the pyramid)

Note that the cranial nerves
VI, VII, and VIII exit in the
groove between the pons
and medulla.

Pons

Pyramid

Atlas Plate VII. Ventral View of the Brain Stem.

98

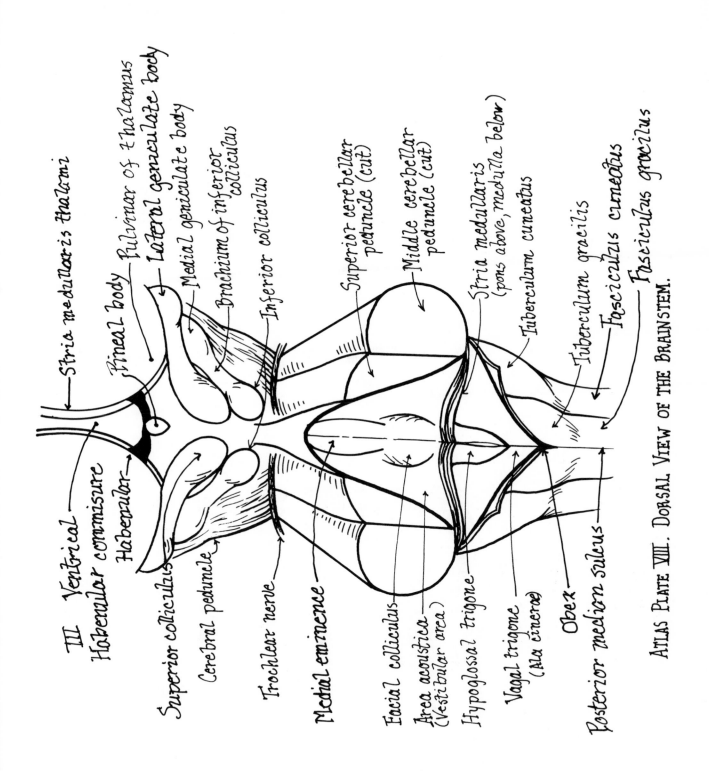

III Ventrical

Habenular commisure

Habenular

Stria medullaris thalami

Pineal body

Pulvinar of thalamus

Lateral geniculate body

Medial geniculate body

Brachium of inferior colliculus

Inferior colliculus

Superior cerebellar peduncle (cut)

Middle cerebellar peduncle (cut)

Stria medullaris (pons above, medulla below)

Tuberculum cuneatus

Tuberculum gracilis

Fasciculus cuneatus

Fasciculus gracilis

Superior colliculus

Cerebral peduncle

Trochlear nerve

Medial eminence

Facial colliculus

Area acoustica (Vestibular area)

Hypoglossal trigone

Vagal trigone (Ala cinerea)

Obex

Posterior median sulcus

ATLAS PLATE VIII. DORSAL VIEW OF THE BRAINSTEM.

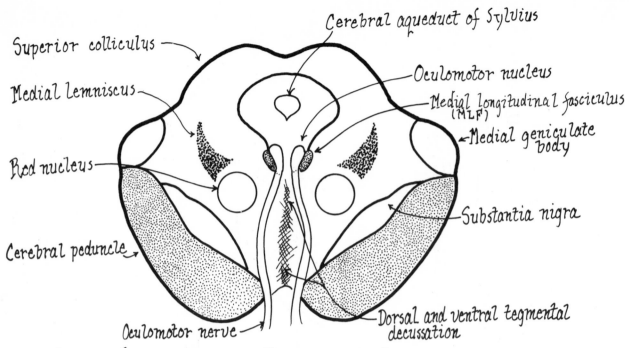

Superior colliculus

Cerebral aqueduct of Sylvius

Medial lemniscus

Oculomotor nucleus

Medial longitudinal fasciculus (MLF)

Red nucleus

Medial geniculate body

Cerebral peduncle

Substantia nigra

Oculomotor nerve

Dorsal and ventral tegmental decussation

ATLAS PLATE IX. CROSS-SECTION OF THE MIDBRAIN AT THE LEVEL OF THE SUPERIOR COLLICULUS.

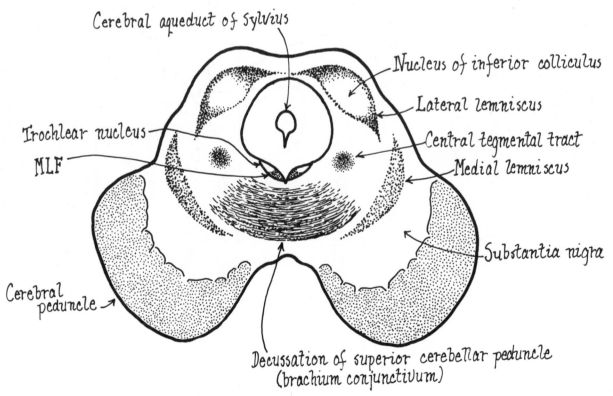

Cerebral aqueduct of Sylvius

Nucleus of inferior colliculus

Lateral lemniscus

Trochlear nucleus

Central tegmental tract

MLF

Medial lemniscus

Substantia nigra

Cerebral peduncle

Decussation of superior cerebellar peduncle (brachium conjunctivum)

ATLAS PLATE X. CROSS-SECTION OF THE MIBRAIN AT THE LEVEL OF THE INFERIOR COLLICULUS.

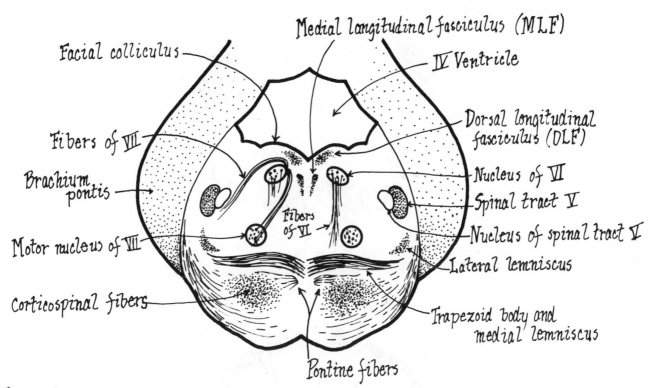

ATLAS PLATE XI. CROSS-SECTION OF THE PONS AT THE FACIAL COLLICULUS.

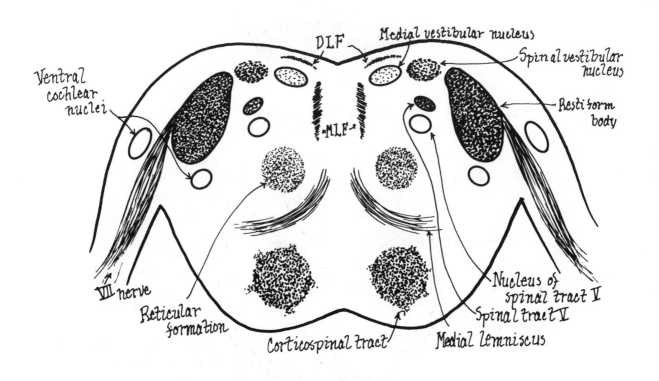

ATLAS PLATE XII. CROSS-SECTION OF LOWER PONS.

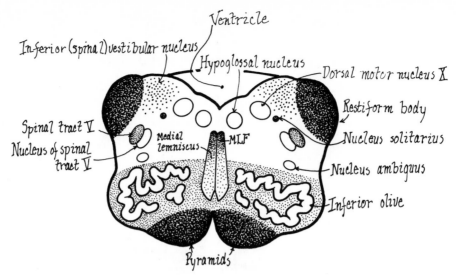

Inferior (spinal) vestibular nucleus

Ventricle

Hypoglossal nucleus

Dorsal motor nucleus X

Restiform body

Spinal tract V

Medial lemniscus

MLF

Nucleus solitarius

Nucleus of spinal tract V

Nucleus ambiguus

Inferior olive

Pyramids

ATLAS PLATE XIII. SECTION THROUGH UPPER MEDULLA.

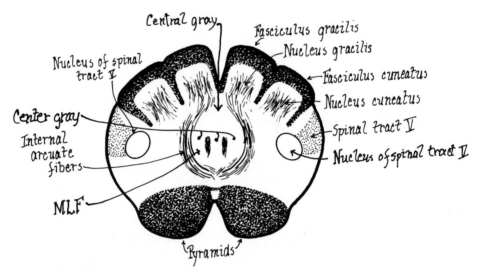

Central gray

Fasciculus gracilis

Nucleus gracilis

Nucleus of spinal tract V

Fasciculus cuneatus

Nucleus cuneatus

Center gray

Spinal tract V

Internal arcuate fibers

Nucleus of spinal tract V

MLF

Pyramids

ATLAS PLATE XIV. SECTION THROUGH LOWER MEDULLA.

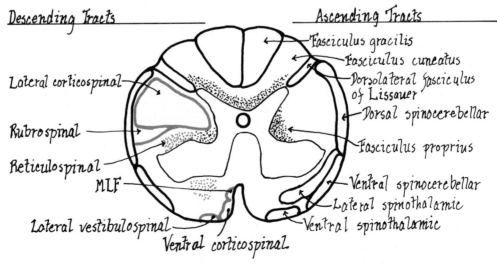

Descending Tracts

Ascending Tracts

Fasciculus gracilis

Lateral corticospinal

Fasciculus cuneatus

Dorsolateral fasciculus of Lissauer

Rubrospinal

Dorsal spinocerebellar

Reticulospinal

Fasciculus proprius

MLF

Ventral spinocerebellar

Lateral vestibulospinal

Lateral spinothalamic

Ventral corticospinal

Ventral spinothalamic

ATLAS PLATE XV. SECTION THROUGH SPINAL CORD AT MIDCERVICAL LEVEL.

EXITING POINTS OF CRANIAL NERVES

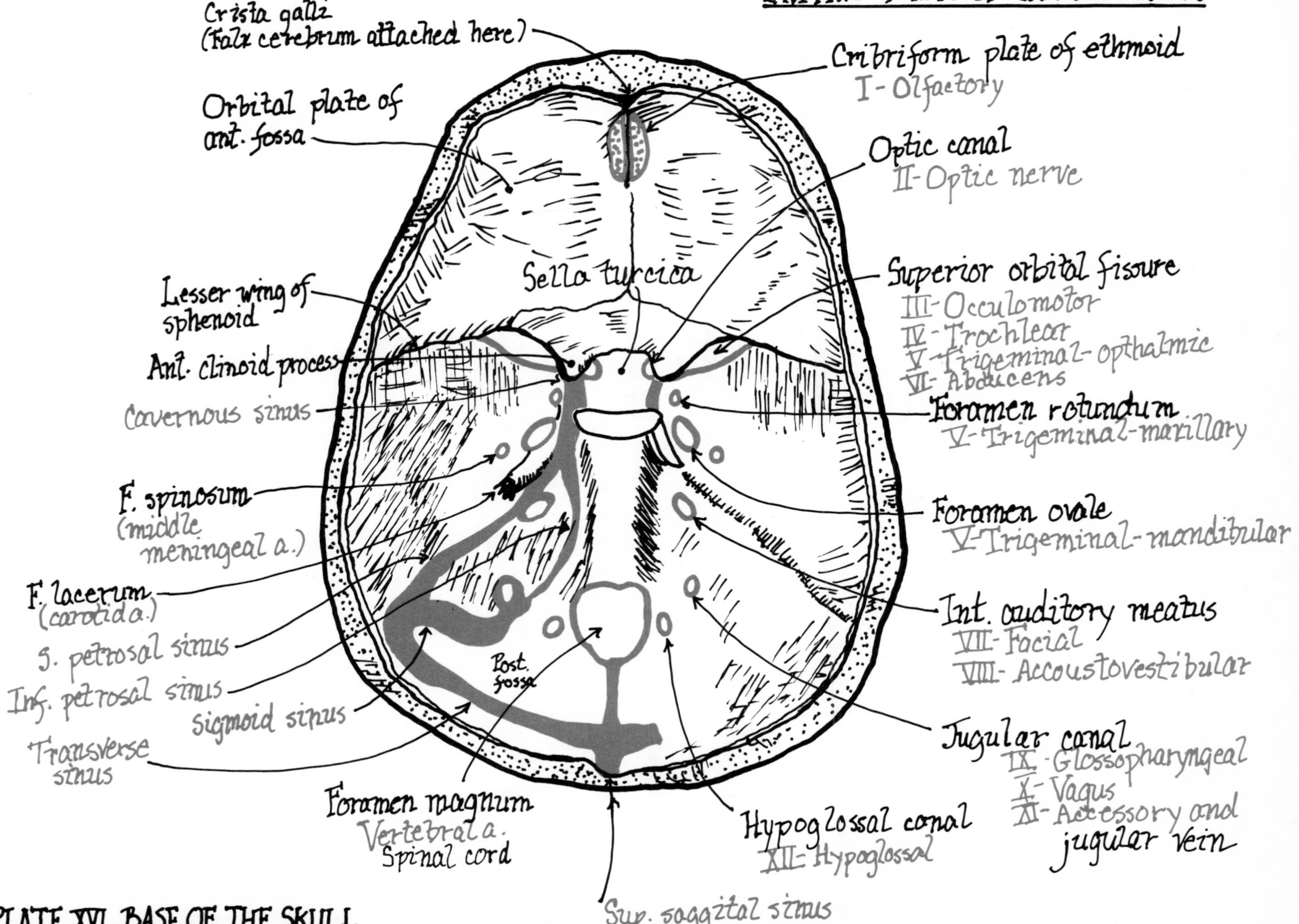

Crista galli
(falx cerebrum attached here)

Orbital plate of
ant. fossa

Cribriform plate of ethmoid
I - Olfactory

Optic canal
II - Optic nerve

Superior orbital fissure
III - Occulomotor
IV - Trochlear
V - Trigeminal - opthalmic
VI - Abducens

Foramen rotundum
V - Trigeminal - maxillary

Foramen ovale
V - Trigeminal - mandibular

Int. auditory meatus
VII - Facial
VIII - Accoustovestibular

Jugular canal
IX - Glossopharyngeal
X - Vagus
XI - Accessory canal
jugular vein

Hypoglossal canal
XII - Hypoglossal

Sup. saggital sinus

Sella turcica

Post.
fossa

Lesser wing of
sphenoid
Ant. clinoid process

Cavernous sinus

F. spinosum
(middle
meningeal a.)

F. lacerum
(carotid a.)

S. petrosal sinus

Inf. petrosal sinus

Sigmoid sinus

Transverse
sinus

Foramen magnum
Vertebral a.
Spinal cord

PLATE XVI. BASE OF THE SKULL

Atlas of Normal and Pathologic Computerized Tomography Scans of the Brain

Prepared by Rina Tadmor, M.D.

The discovery of x-rays by William Roentgen in 1895 was one of the great contributions to medicine. A further revolutionary step was made in 1972 by the physicist Godfrey Hounsfield and the neuroradiologist James Ambrose, who introduced the technique of computerized tomography (CT). They, like Roentgen, won the Nobel Prize in Medicine for their work.

In conventional radiology, most of the shadows and outlines of the various three-dimensional structures are superimposed on a two-dimensional film. Further, in conventional x-rays of the skull, the brain is not seen because of its low density. However, CT is about 100 times more sensitive than conventional radiography and enables one to see clearly the brain and its subdivisions. CT images appear in the various shades of gray from black to white. In the negative mode (the one most commonly used in CT) the densest objects and materials, such as bone, appear as white, whereas those of low density, such as cerebrospinal fluid, are black. The ventricular system, the cerebral sulci, and similar structures are thus rendered quite visible. This mode of presenting the CT image may at first present some confusion, as the gray matter in the basal ganglia, cerebral cortex, and elsewhere appears white on a CT scan, because it is packed with cell bodies and is therefore relatively dense. The white matter is lower in density and therefore shows up as gray or black.

A complete CT examination of the brain involves 10–12 successive, parallel, horizontal scans or "cuts" of the brain. The injection of intravenous contrast substances enhances the visibility of lesions and thereby facilitates the viewing of such pathologic conditions as tumors and abscesses.

This atlas provides a basic understanding of normal and abnormal CT scans. With this foundation, the student can go on to further reading and practice interpreting more detailed scans. Figures 1–4 in this atlas are normal horizontal scans. The drawing on this page indicates the level at which each cut was taken. The ventricular system is outlined in red in the drawing; it appears in black in the CT images themselves. Figure 5 is a coronal scan, and Figures 6 and 7 are partial horizontal scans showing the orbital areas and the structures of the ear, respectively. The eleven pathologic scans in Figures 8–18 represent some of the most common disease conditions seen in the neurologic service.

Finally, listed below are three important works related to CT that will give you a deeper understanding of this very important subject:

Kieffer, S. A., and Heitzman, E. R., *Atlas of Cross-Sectional Computed Tomography, Ultrasound, Radiography, Gross Anatomy.* Harper & Row, New York, 1979.

Harwood-Nash, D. C., *Neuroradiology in Infants and Children*, Volume II, pp. 461–504. C. V. Mosby, St. Louis, 1976.

Gonzales, C. F., Grossman, C., and Palacios, J., *Computed Brain and Orbital Tomography: Technique and Interpretation.* John Wiley & Sons, New York, 1976.

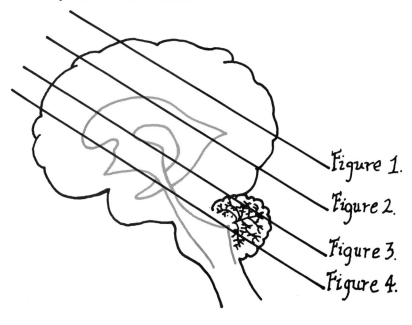

Figure 1.

Figure 2.

Figure 3.

Figure 4.

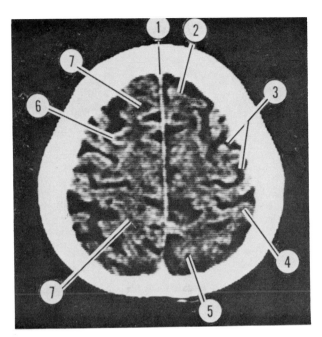

Figure 1. Horizontal section of the superior part of the normal brain.

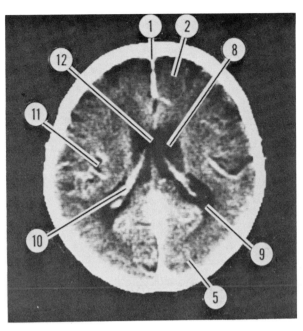

Figure 2. Horizontal (axial) section at a lower (inferior) level.

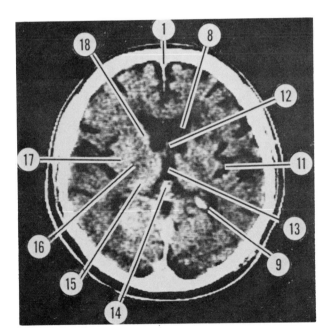

Figure 3. Horizontal section at a still lower level.

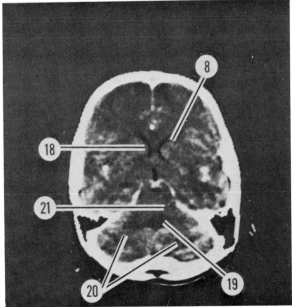

Figure 4. Horizontal section through the basal part of the brain.

Legend: *1*, falx cerebrum; *2*, frontal lobe; *3*, sulcus; *4*, gyrus; *5*, occipital lobe; *6*, gray matter; *7*, white matter; *8*, anterior horn of lateral ventricle; *9*, posterior horn of lateral ventricle; *10*, choroid plexus; *11*, insula; *12*, septum pellucidum; *13*, third ventricle; *14*, calcified pineal body; *15*, thalamus; *16*, internal capsule; *17*, lentiform nucleus; *18*, head of caudate nucleus; *19*, fourth ventricle; *20*, cerebellar hemisphere; *21*, pons.

Several of the illustrations in this section were provided courtesy of the Elscint Corporation and are reproduced with their permission.

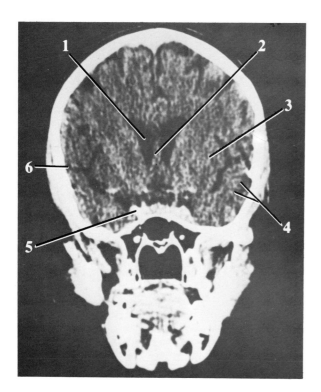

Figure 5. Coronal section of the brain 1 inch anterior to the external auditory meatus. *1*, lateral ventricle; *2*, septum pellucidum; *3*, insula; *4*, temporal lobe; *5*, cavernous sinus; *6*, lateral fissure.

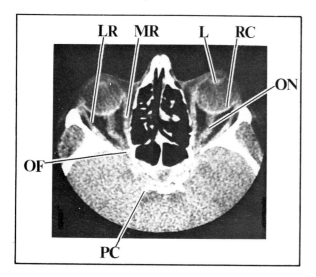

Figure 6. Horizontal cut through the middle of the orbits. *L*, lens; *RC*, retina and choroid; *ON*, optic nerve; *LR*, lateralis rectus muscle; *MR*, medial rectus muscle; *OF*, optic foramen; *PC*, posterior clinoid process of the sella turcica.

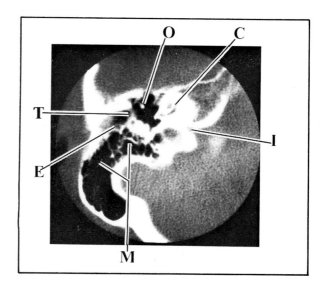

Figure 7. Horizontal section through the middle and inner ear. *E*, external auditory canal; *T*, tympanic membrane (eardrum); *O*, ossicle in middle ear cavity; *C*, cochlea in inner ear cavity; *I*, internal auditory canal; *M*, mastoid air cells.

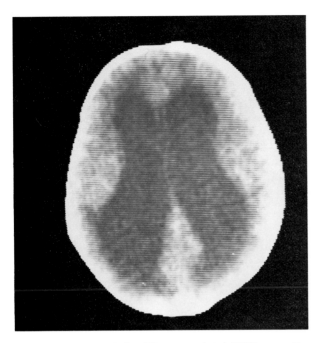

Figure 8. Hydrocephalus. The accumulated CSF has greatly increased the size of the lateral ventricles.

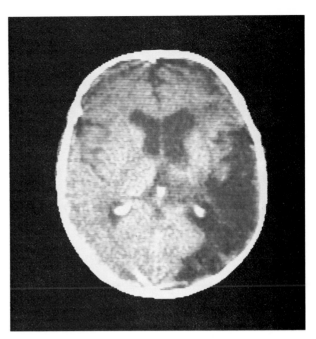

Figure 9. Infarct. Obstruction of the right middle cerebral artery has produced a dark infarcted area in the parieto-occipital lobes with no displacement of brain structures. Nondisplacement is typical in infarcts due to emboli and thrombi. The three white spots are the capillary-rich choroid plexus filled with contrast medium.

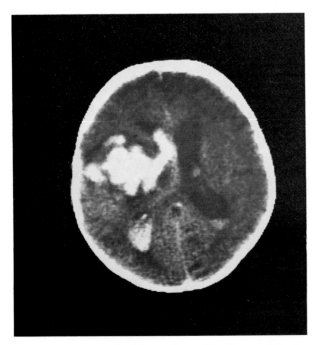

Figure 10. Intracerebral hemorrhage. The dense, white, irregular mass in the left parietal lobe represents blood, which has also ruptured into the lateral ventricle and caused displacement of structures. Displacement will occur in all space-occupying lesions.

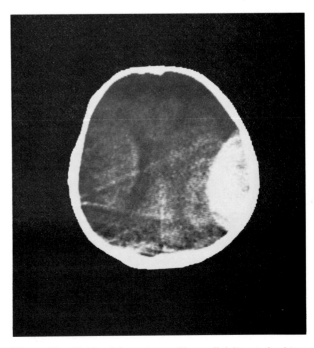

Figure 11. Epidural hematoma. The well-delineated white area represents an extracerebral hemorrhage in the right parietal region, causing compression and closure of the lateral ventricle on the same side.

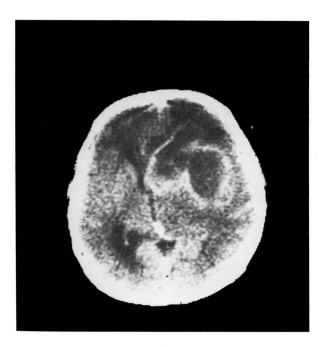

Figure 12. Abscess. A multilobulated mass in the frontoparietal lobes has caused massive displacement of brain tissues and structure. Abscesses can only be differentiated from gliomas (Figure 14) on the basis of clinical and laboratory findings.

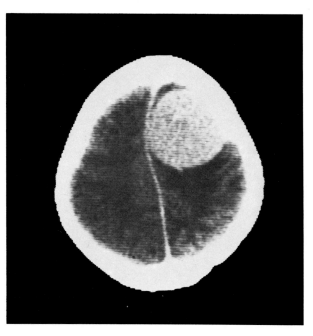

Figure 13. Meningioma. The round, white, homogeneous tumor in the right frontal lobe has caused a displacement of the falx cerebrum. The whiteness, homogeneity, and roundness are quite typical of meningiomas.

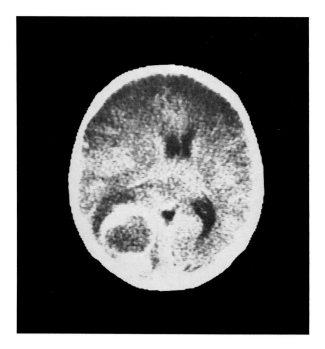

Figure 14. Astrocytoma. This round, well-delineated, nonhomogeneous tumor in the left parieto-occipital lobes is surrounded by a dark edematous area. This growth has caused a shift in structures as seen by the displaced septum pellucidum and obliteration of the posterior horn of the lateral ventricle.

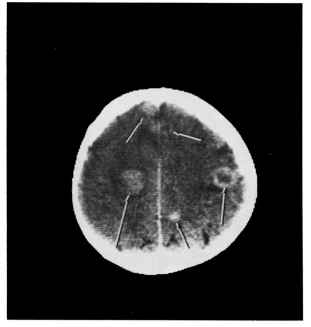

Figure 15. Metastasis. Multiple round lesions (arrows) in both hemispheres represent metastatic spread ("seeding") from a primary tumor elsewhere in the body. The white ring, characteristic of various nonspecific lesions (e.g., tumors, abscesses, fungal diseases) indicates a breakdown of the blood-brain barrier.

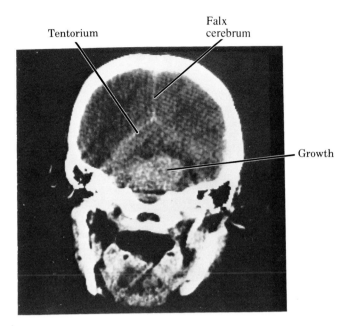

Figure 16. A CT coronal study of the posterior fossa following intravenous contrast injections showing the falx and tentorium and a hyperdense lesion occupying most of the posterior fossa with surrounding edema (black halo), most probably a medulloblastoma.

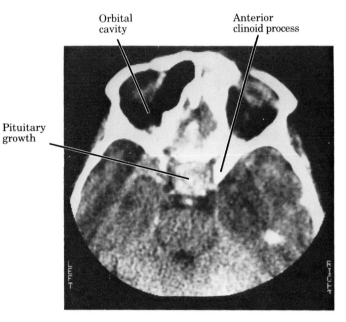

Figure 17. A horizontal section of the head at the level of the sella turcica showing a pituitary growth.

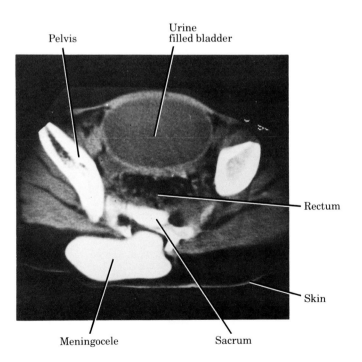

Figure 18. CT Myelography. Cross section of the pelvis of a child showing spina bifida of the sacrum with a meningocele located beneath the skin but not forming a protruding sac.

Normal and Pathologic Magnetic Resonance Scans of the Brain

Prepared by Rina Tadmor, M.D.

Magnetic resonance imaging (MRI) is a form of imaging modality based on the interaction of a magnet, radiofrequency energy, and the protons of molecules. The data obtained are then fed into a computer, and the result is seen as an image on a screen. Because hydrogen is present in all tissues, as well as other considerations, it has been chosen for imaging, (i.e., the proton of the hydrogen atom is the one that is measured). However, it is possible to use the protons of other atoms, such as carbon or magnesium, for imaging purposes.

MRI's advantages over CT scanning are that it doesn't require the use of ionizing radiation and it is also much more sensitive, thus allowing the visualization of smaller anatomic structures and de-tails. It also permits imaging to be done in the sagittal plane. It should be noted however that, because the proton density of hydrogen in bone and calcified tissue is low, their visualization is poor and thus details in or about them can be missed. It seems at present that MRI will not replace CT and other imaging techniques but in the near future will be a complementary examination, the choice being dictated on a case-by-case basis. Because spectroscopy is another option available by MRI, it will be a potentially valuable tool in research.

It is the author's intention to present the reader with introductory pictures of normal MR scans and some simple pathologic scans in order to familiarize him or her with this new imaging modality.

Note: The basic theoretical work was done in the 1940s by the American physicists Felix Bloch and Edward Purcell who in 1952 won the Nobel Prize for their work.

All pictures were taken on the Elscint Gyrex S-5000 and Gyrex 2T. The authors wish to thank the Elscint Corporation for the use of these scans and for their generous assistance.

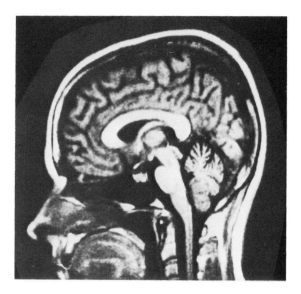

Figure 1a.   Midsagittal section of the brain.

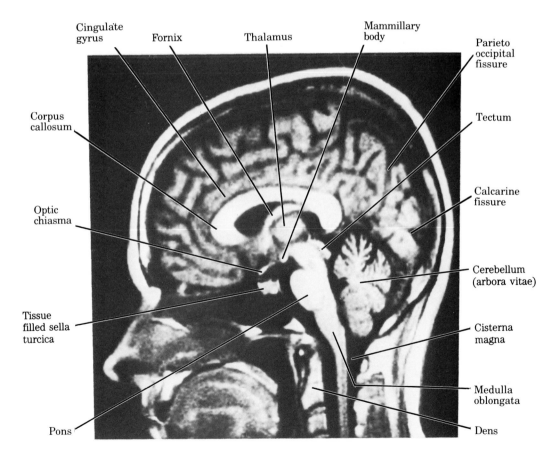

Figure 1b.   Midsagittal section of the brain with identifying leaders.

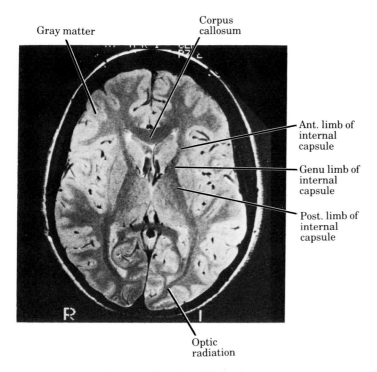

Figure 2. Horizontal section of the brain.

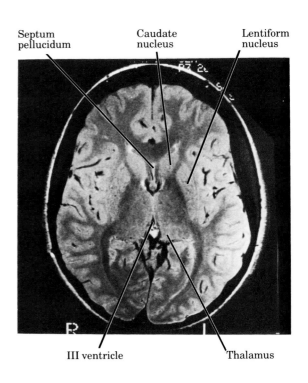

Figure 3. A horizontal section of the brain, lower (more caudal) than Figure 2.

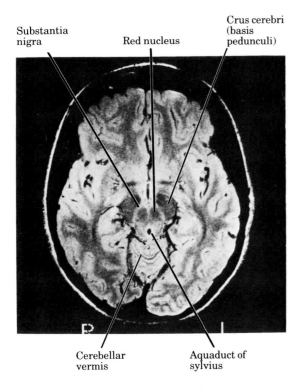

Figure 4. A horizontal section of the brain lower than Figures 2 and 3 showing the midbrain.

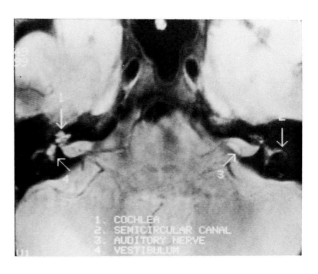

Figure 5. MRI scan of the inner ear.

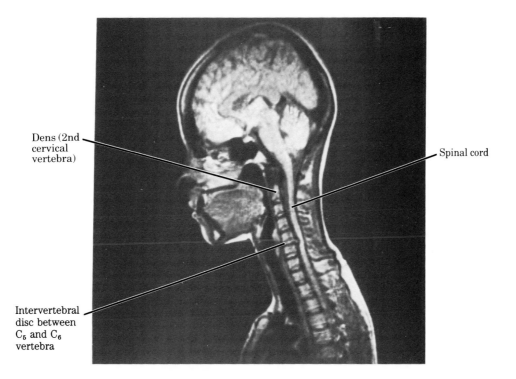

Dens (2nd
cervical
vertebra)

Spinal cord

Intervertebral
disc between
C₅ and C₆
vertebra

Figure 6.   Midsagittal MRI scan of the spinal cord showing a
"slipped" disc which is impinging on the cord in the cervical
region.

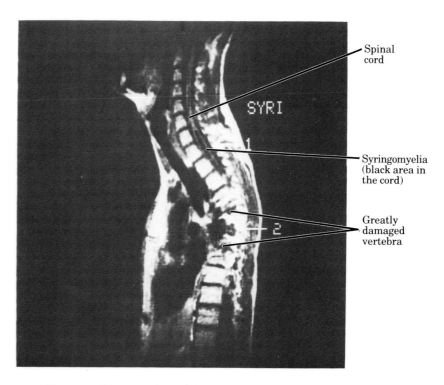

Spinal
cord

SYRI

Syringomyelia
(black area in
the cord)

Greatly
damaged
vertebra

Figure 7.   Syringomyelia and damaged thoracic vertebra.

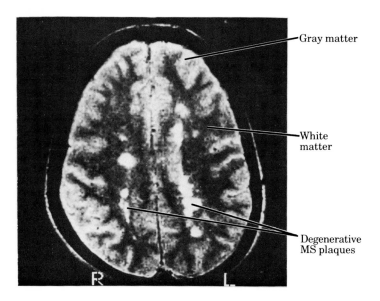

Figure 8. Multiple Sclerosis. Horizontal section of the cerebral hemispheres showing degenerative plaques in the white matter which is black on the picture.

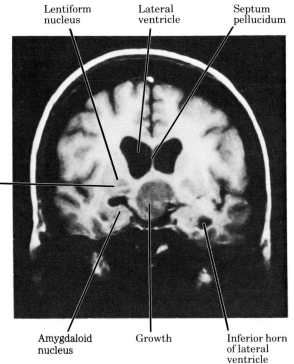

Figure 9. Coronal section of the brain at the level of the anterior commissure showing a growth at the base of brain (also see Plate V, Appendix II for orientation).

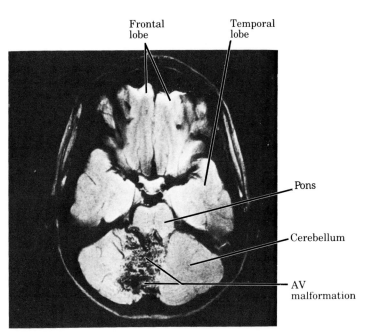

Figure 10. AV malformation. The black area in the cerebellum represents a mass of arteries and veins.

Sample Examination Questions

1. Which of the following tracts or pathways is completely uncrossed in its entire course?
   a. Pain and temperature from the face
   b. Proprioception from the body
   c. Corticospinal
   d. Dorsal spinocerebellar
   e. Vestibular pathways
2. What condition results if the right optic nerve is cut?
   a. Left homonymous hemianopsia
   b. Bitemporal hemianopsia
   c. Right homonymous hemianopsia
   d. Binasal hemianopsia
   e. None of the above
3. Which of the following is not true concerning the hypothalamus?
   a. It is concerned with temperature regulation
   b. It has a hunger center
   c. It is concerned with equilibrium
   d. It influences pituitary secretions
   e. It has areas concerned with emotional reactions
4. Which of the following statements concerning the neuron is not true?
   a. It is very sensitive to oxygen deprivation
   b. If the axon is cut the cell body will always die
   c. Myelin is laid down by the sheath of Schwann in the PNS
   d. Nissl bodies are found in the cytoplasm of the cell body
   e. Mature neurons don't undergo mitosis
5. Which of the following tracts doesn't synapse on the final common pathway?
   a. Rubrospinal tract
   b. Corticospinal tract
   c. Spinothalamic tract
   d. Vestibulospinal tract
   e. All of the above
6. Which of the following is not a sign of cerebellar injury?
   a. Uncoordinated movements
   b. Dizziness
   c. Athetosis
   d. Falling
   e. Intention tremor

In the following three questions match the tract with the peduncle in which it runs:

7. Corticopontocerebellar tract
8. Dentorubrothalamic tract
9. Vestibulocerebellar tract
   a. Superior cerebellar peduncle
   b. Middle cerebellar peduncle
   c. Inferior cerebellar peduncle
10. Obstruction of the left anterior cerebral artery past the anterior communicating artery is likely to cause defective movement or paralysis in the:
    a. Right lower limb
    b. Right upper limb
    c. Muscles of the face on the left side
    d. Muscles of the face on the right side
    e. Left lower limb

11. With respect to the subcortical motor areas (i.e., basal ganglia, etc.) all of the following statements are true except:
    a. Damage to them can result in pill-rolling tremor
    b. They aren't connected to the cerebral cortex
    c. They are part of the extrapyramidal system
    d. They are connected with the red nucleus
    e. They are connected with the thalamus

12. A patient exhibits bitemporal hemianopsia. In which of the following areas is the lesion most likely to be?
    a. Lateral geniculate body
    b. Midline of the optic chiasma
    c. Optic radiations
    d. Visual cortex
    e. Optic tract

13. Which of the following don't synapse in the thalamus?
    a. Pain and temperature from the face
    b. Fibers from the dentate nucleus
    c. Proprioception fibers from the body
    d. Auditory fibers
    e. Pressure and touch fibers from the face

14. A patient suffers from an upper neuron paralysis that affects the arm. The lesion can be in any of the following areas except:
    a. Motor cortex
    b. Internal capsule
    c. Crus cerebri (basis pedunculi)
    d. Tegmentum of the midbrain
    e. Pyramid
    f. Lateral white column of the spinal cord

15. If the dorsal spinal root is cut in the sacral region, which of the following would show Wallerian degeneration in the cervical area of the cord?
    a. Spinothalamic tract
    b. Fasciculus cuneatus
    c. Ventral spinocerebellar tract
    d. Lateral corticospinal tract
    e. Fasciculus gracilis

16. The cell bodies of the preganglionic parasympathetic fibers that innervate the descending colon are situated in the:
    a. Dorsal motor nucleus of the vagus
    b. Nucleus ambiguus
    c. Lateral gray column of the spinal cord in the thoracic segments T_{10}–T_{12}
    d. Inferior mesenteric ganglion
    e. Lateral gray column of the spinal cord in the S_2–S_4 sacral segments

17. A patient has total deafness in the left ear. In which of the following areas is the lesion most likely to be?
    a. Left superior temporal gyrus
    b. Right and left cochlear nuclei
    c. Left auditory nerve
    d. Left lateral lemniscus
    e. Right and left inferior colliculi

18. Examination reveals that a patient doesn't sweat in the area supplied by thoracic spinal nerves T_1–T_2. A lesion in which area won't give rise to this condition?
    a. Sympathetic trunk
    b. Intermediate lateral gray column of the spinal cord
    c. Ventral roots of the spinal cord

   d. White rami communicantes

   e. Dorsal roots of spinal nerve

   f. Gray rami communicantes

In the following three questions three common reflexes are listed. Match them with the correct cranial nerves that are involved in the reflex arc.

19. Corneal reflex
20. Horizontal nystagmus
21. Gag reflex
   a. optic-facial
   b. vestibular-facial
   c. glossopharyngeal-vagus
   d. vestibular-oculomotor and abducens
   e. trigeminal-facial
   f. trigeminal-vagus

Answer the following questions by indicating the letter of the statement that correctly applies.
   a. If both statements are true and there is a causal relationship between the two
   b. If both statements are true but there is no causal relationship between the two
   c. If the first statement is true but the second is false
   d. If the first statement is false and the second is true
   e. If both statements are false

22. Most of the spinocerebellar fibers enter the cerebellum on the ipsilateral side, and therefore injury to the right inferior cerebellar peduncle results in a person falling to the right side.
23. Damage to the genu of the left internal capsule results in a paralysis of the entire right side of the face, because the corticobulbar fibers are located in the genu of the internal capsule.
24. If the right thalamus is damaged then the patient will lose all somatic sensations on the left side of the body and face, because these fibers all eventually cross over to the opposite side from which they entered the cord and brainstem.

ANSWERS

1. *d*	6. *c*	11. *b*	16. *e*	21. *c*
2. *e*	7. *b*	12. *b*	17. *c*	22. *a*
3. *c*	8. *a*	13. *d*	18. *e*	23. *d*
4. *b*	9. *c*	14. *d*	19. *e*	24. *e*
5. *c*	10. *a*	15. *e*	20. *d*	

Relax With "Did You Know?" "Ten Greatest Discoveries," and "Odds and Ends"

DID YOU KNOW?

. . . That in order to study medicine in England the first woman had to disguise herself as a man! "Dr. James Barry kept the secret of her sex all her life and had a successful career in the British Army where she was honored for distinguished service during the Battle of Waterloo. Only after her death in 1865 was her true sex and the fact that she had had a child revealed" (Taylor, A. The female doctor's dilemma. *Illustrated London News.* 271: p. 45. Dec. 1983. Ms. Taylor has also informed the author that more about Dr. Barry can be found in *Women in History: Thirty-Five Centuries of Feminine Achievement* by Susan Raven and Alison Weir, published by Weidenfeld & Nicholson.

* * *

. . . That placing the cold water knob on the right side and the hot one on the left side of the water basin has a neuroanatomic basis! Most people (95%) are right-handed and instinctively reach out for and turn the knob on the right side. Therefore, in order to prevent inadvertent scalding the right side controls the cold water. True, you left-handed people are being discriminated against, but you've always been treated with suspicion and disdain. The word "sinister" means left-sided in Latin, and honored guests are always seated on the right side of the host. Until recently left-handed children were often forced to learn to write with the right hand until it was discovered that this often produced great inner turmoil that was frequently expressed by stammering.

* * *

. . . That the philosophers Maimonides and William James, and the authors Chekhov, John Keats, Somerset Maugham, and Sir Arthur Conan Doyle, the creator of Sherlock Holmes, were all physicians. Benjamin Rush, a signer of the Declaration of Independence, as well as the inventor of the guillotine, Dr. Guillotine, were also renowned physicians.

* * *

. . . That for centuries, the bodies of executed criminals were used for dissection. In Edinburgh in 1725 the body of Maggie Dickson "came back to life" shortly after she was hanged and before the medical students had a chance to get at it. She continued to live for many years afterwards and was known as "Half-Hanged Maggie Dickson."

* * *

. . . Oedipus had swollen feet! (that should have been his only problem). Being told that his infant son would grow up and kill him, his father bound Oedipus' ankles and placed him on a mountainside to die. There, a wandering shepherd found him with his feet swollen by the tight rope. He adopted the unknown babe and named him Edepes after his most prominent feature, (i.e., his swollen feet). "Ede-" in Greek means swollen, from which is derived the word edema, and "pes" or "ped" means feet, as in pedestrian, pedal, and pes hippocampus.

* * *

. . . That the red-and-white striped barber pole is a trademark of surgeons. In the Middle Ages, barbers, not physicians, did surgery, and to indicate their place of business to the general population who couldn't read, they displayed their sign outside their shops—a pole with a red stripe symbolizing blood and a white one symbolizing bandages.

* * *

. . . That percussion, the technique of tapping the chest to diagnose conditions by the nature of the sound response, was discovered by Dr. Auenbrugger. The idea came to him from having watched his father, a tavern keeper, tap on beer kegs to determine the extent to which they were full.

* * *

. . . That one of the co-discoverers of insulin didn't share the Nobel Prize because he was only a medical student! In June of 1921, Dr. Banting, a surgical resident and George Best, a third-year medical student at McGill University, were reluctantly given a small, run-down laboratory in which to do their research by Dr. McCloud, who then went away on his summer holiday. In 3 months at work, the two extracted and identified insulin from the pancreas. The Nobel Committee, however, awarded their prize to Banting and McCloud, and overlooked Best because he was still only a medical student. Banting, however, showed his true worth and opinion by publicly sharing his half of the prize with Best.

* * *

...That the British are called "limies" because for over 200 years their sailors were required to drink lime juice to prevent scurvy, a disease caused by vitamin C deficiency.

* * *

...That the words "testify" and all its derivatives (e.g., testimony, testate) come from the word "testicle." In ancient Roman courts only men were allowed to give evidence. In order to prevent a women from disguising herself as a man and giving evidence, all witnesses had to come before the judge to prove to him that they were male by lifting their togas and revealing their testicles. This isn't as strange as it sounds; in today's Olympic games women have to prove they are female by passing both a physical and chromosomal examination. This testing is done because a few years ago one of the Great Powers managed to smuggle men disguised as women into the track and field events (especially discus, shotput, and javelin).

* * *

...That gauze was invented by the Arabs and named after the city where it was produced—Gaza.

* * *

...That Jenner got the idea for vaccination from a dairy maid who told him, "I can't get smallpox since I've already had cowpow" (the latter is a mild form of smallpox).

* * *

...That dice were, for centuries, carved from animal bones and the crapshooter today still uses the expression, "Roll them bones."

* * *

...That Pare, the great French surgeon, introduced ligatures. Until the 16th century hemorrhage from sword or gunshot wounds was stopped by applying a hot poker or boiling oil to the wound. As late as 1870 antiseptic technique was unknown, and surgeons while operating kept the sutures in the buttonholes of their vests or jackets!

TEN GREATEST DISCOVERIES

Most of us like lists so here's one on the ten greatest discoveries in modern medicine, arranged in chronological order. From Dr. William Roentgen (number 4) on, each of the discoveries mentioned resulted in a Nobel Prize.

1. General Anesthesia

In 1842, Dr. Crawford Long, a country general practitioner in Georgia, first started using ether as a general anesthetic in his practice, but he didn't publish his work until 1849. Meanwhile working independently in New England, Drs. Morton and Wells, and C. T. Jackson, a pharmacist, also discovered ether's anesthetic properties in 1846. Later that year it was used for the first time at Massachusetts General Hospital, and from there its use spread rapidly throughout the world.

2. Germs as the Cause of Disease

From 1860–1870, Louis Pasteur, a French biochemist, discovered and laid down the facts that form the basis of bacteriology and microbiology—"the germ theory." In addition, he discovered the vaccine against rabies, as well as the process of heating such substances as milk to kill pathologic microorganisms, pasteurization.

3. Antiseptic Technique

Before 1876, physicians would operate in their streetclothes with the surgical sutures kept in the buttonholes of their jackets or vests and pulled out as needed!! Then in that year Lord Lister of England proposed and used in his operations sterile, antiseptic techniques. As a result, his mortality rates dropped from 45 to 15%, which is very good considering the fact that there were no antibiotics, adrenalin, etc. and they didn't know about fluid replacement and acid-base balance.

4. X-Rays

In November 1895, Dr. William Roentgen, a German physicist, discovered x-rays and announced his findings, and within a year more than a thousand papers on this new diagnostic technique were published throughout the world. One English newspaper even ran an ad for special underwear that guaranteed to "keep the private parts private" during an x-ray examination.

5. Discovery of Blood Groups

Blood transfusions from sheep to humans and from human to human were tried by Robert Boyle and others as early as 1667, but were banned when some of the patients died following the procedure. It wasn't until 1903 that Karl Landsteiner of the Rockefeller Institute discovered the four major blood groups that explained compatibility and incompatibility and thus permitted safe transfusions. In 1940 Landsteiner, working with Dr. Wiener, discovered the Rh-factor.

6. Discovery of Insulin

In ten weeks of research during the summer of 1921, Dr. Banting, a second-year surgical resident who had never done any research, and Charles Best, a third-year medical student, discovered insulin and later used it successfully for the first time on a dying diabetic patient. Dr. Banting won the Nobel Prize, but the Nobel Committee refused to give it to Best because he was only a student. Incidentally they worked in a run-down laboratory and used ten dogs for their work.

7. The Isolation of and the Role Played by Neurotransmitters

During the 1920s, Sir Henry Dale in England and Otto Lowie in Germany did a series of simple yet brilliant experiments in which they discovered acetylcholine and epinephrine and demonstrated their function as neurotransmitters.

8. Antibiotics

In 1927 Alexander Fleming, an English researcher accidently left open a petri dish of *Staphylococcus* that he was culturing. Returning several days later he noticed that the colonies of cocci were being destroyed by a mold, and this led him to investigate the mold—penicillin notatum. However he didn't follow up the therapeutic implications of this finding, and it was not until 1940 that Chain and Florey at Oxford did so and published their findings in a three-page report in *Lancet*. Finally in 1948 Waxman discovered the broad-spectrum antibiotic streptomycin.

9. DNA

The work of Watson and Crick on DNA in the early 1950s opened the door to the age of molecular biology, modern genetics, and all their off shoots.

Note: Some may ask, "How about vaccination," but this is a very old technique that was understood and used by Dr. Jenner in the 18th century. He noted that milkmaids didn't get smallpox because they had already been infected by a milder form, known as cowpox. On this observation he based his successful therapy of inoculation.

10. Computerized Tomography (CT) and Magnetic Resonance Imaging (MRI)

As mentioned previously the physicists Godfrey Hounsfield and the neuroradiologist James Ambrose discovered computerized tomography, while the physicists Bloch and Purcell performed the theoretical work that led to the use of magnetic resonance imaging.

ODDS AND ENDS

Henri de Mondeville was a renowned 14th-century doctor. Perhaps part of his fame was due to his method of supporting his patients—"Keep up your patient's spirit by music....or by giving him forged letters describing the death of his enemy."

* * *

Quarantine come from the Italian word "quarante" meaning 40, the number of days a suspected person was isolated.

* * *

Rhazes, the great Persian doctor (841–926), in choosing a site for a hospital, hung fresh meat in different parts of the city and selected that place where the meat had spoiled the least.

* * *

The symbol for male, ♂, is the arrow of Mars the god of war, whereas the one for female ♀ represents the handmirror of Venus.

* * *

We complain about overspecialization in medicine but listen to this: "The practice of medicine is so divided that each physician is a healer of one disease and no more, some of the eye, some of the teeth and some of the belly." This was written 2,500 years by the Greek historian Herodotus who visited Egypt and described the situation there. One doctor had the glorious title "Shepherd of the Anus," and I imagine that Johnny Carson or a gag writer could really "take off" on this.

* * *

Today in Russia there are more women doctors than male physicians. In the United States women make up 30–35% of those entering medical schools, but this percentage was not always so high. Twenty years ago only 8–10% of medical students were women. The first medical school in America was founded in Philadelphia in 1765, but it wasn't until 1850 that the first medical school for women was opened—the Women's Medical College of Pennsylvania in Philadelphia.

*   *   *

The symbol R$_x$ on prescriptions comes from ancient Egypt. Originally it was shaped 𝓡 and represented the Eye of Horus, the god of protection and recovery.

*   *   *

The ancient Egyptian treatment for baldness consisted of spreading a mixture made out of the fat of the lion, the hippo, the deer, and the crocodile; one medical historian commented that the Egyptian pharmacy schools must have had hunting as part of their curriculum! We know so much about ancient Egyptian medicine via two papyri—the Smith and Ebers that are named after their discoverers and that date back 3,600 years.

*   *   *

Sterile wax is used in neurosurgical operations to staunch bleeding from the skull bones.

*   *   *

Migraine is a corruption of the French words "hemi-crain" meaning half the head. Over a period of time the first two letters "he" were dropped, leaving the word "micrain", or as is spelled now, "migraine."

*   *   *

Bedside teaching of students was popular in ancient Rome, but the writer Martial poked fun at it in this verse:

"I called you Dr. Symmachus for a
slight indisposition.
You brought your hundred students
as befits a real clinician.
With hands all chilled by winters blasts,
they practiced their palpatation.
The fever that I didn't have
is now a conflagration."

Index